Trauma: Who cares?

A report of the National Confidential Enquiry into Patient Outcome and Death (2007)

Compiled by:

G Findlay MB ChB FRCA

I C Martin LLM FRCS FDSRCS

S Carter MBBS FRCS FRCS(G) RCPS

N Smith BS

D Weyman

M Mason F

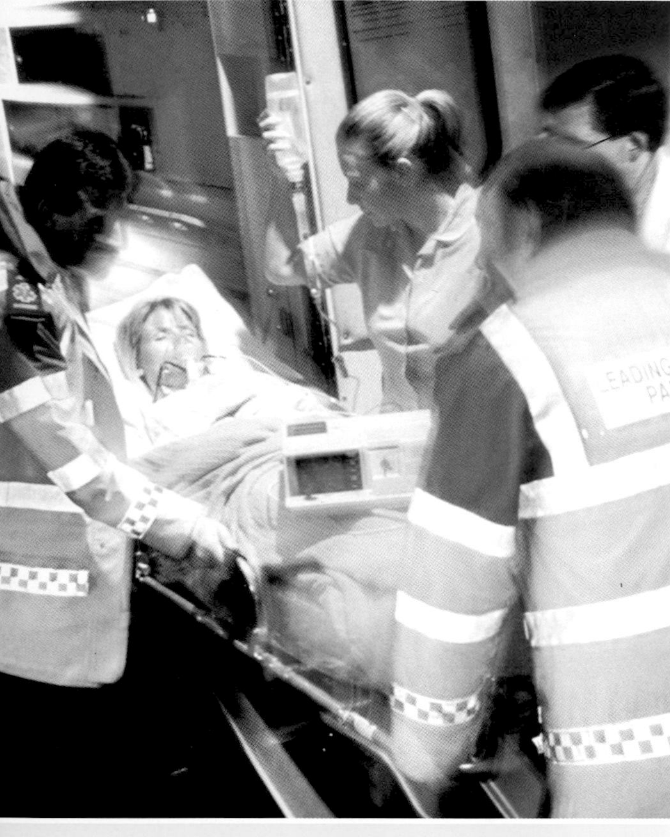

Contents

Acknowledgements

This is the twenty first report published by NCEPOD and, as always, could not have been achieved without the support of a wide range of individuals and organisations. Our particular thanks go to:

The Expert Group who advised NCEPOD:

Dr B Winter
Consultant in Adult Critical Care

Dr C Carney
Chief Executive East Anglian Ambulance NHS Trust

Mr D Gilroy
Consultant General Surgeon

Mr Keith Porter
Consultant Orthopaedic Surgeon

Professor P Giannoudis
Professor of Trauma and Orthopaedics

Mr S Davies
Trauma Nurse Co-ordinator

Professor T Coats
Professor of Emergency Medicine

Mr T Pigott
Consultant Spinal Surgeon

Ms E Symonds
Lay Representative

Dr A Gray
Consultant Anaesthetist

The Advisors who reviewed the cases:

Dr A Wilson
Consultant in Emergency Medicine

Miss A Hutchings
Nurse

Dr A Feazey
Consultant in Emergency Medicine

Dr A Black
Consultant Paediatrician

Miss A McGinley
Nurse

Dr A Sutcliffe
Consultant in Intensive Care

Mr A Armstrong
Consultant Plastic Surgeon

Mr B White
Consultant Neurosurgeon

Dr C Stevenson
Specialist Registrar in Anaesthesia

Dr C Gomez
Consultant in Intensive Care

Dr C Deakin
Consultant Anaesthetist

Dr D Gardiner
Consultant in Intensive Care

Dr D Bryden
Consultant in Intensive Care

Mr D Teanby
Consultant Orthopaedic Surgeon

Dr D Esberger
Consultant in Emergency Medicine

Dr E Abrahamson
Consultant in Emergency Medicine

Miss H Cattermole
Consultant Orthopaedic Surgeon

Dr J Berridge
Consultant Anaesthetist

Mr K Brohi
Consultant General Surgeon

Major M Butler
Specialist Registrar in Trauma and Orthopaedics

Mr M Perry
Consultant Oral and Maxillofacial Surgeon

Mr M McMonagle
Specialist Registrar in General Surgery

Mr N Tai
Consultant Vascular Surgeon

Dr O Bagshaw
Consultant Paediatrician

Dr R Landau
Consultant in Emergency Medicine

Dr R Banks
Specialist Registrar in Maxillofacial Surgery

Mr S Marks
Consultant Neurosurgeon

Dr S Smith
Consultant in Emergency Medicine

Dr S Luney
Consultant Anaesthetist

Acknowledgements

The organisations that provided funding to cover the cost of this study:

National Patient Safety Agency
Department of Health, Social Services and Public Safety (Northern Ireland)
Aspen Healthcare
Benenden Hospital
BMI Healthcare
BUPA
Capio Group
Covenant Healthcare
Cromwell Hospital
Isle of Man Health and Social Security Department
Fairfield Independent Hospital
HCA International
Horder Centre
Hospital Management Trust
Hospital of St John and St Elizabeth
King Edward VII Hospital
King Edward VIIs Hospital Sister Agnes
London Clinic
McIndoe Surgical Centre
Mount Alvernia Hospital
Netcare Healthcare
New Victoria Hospital
North Wales Medical Centre
Nuffield Hospitals
Orchard Hospital
St Anthony's Hospital
St Joseph's Hospital
Spencer Wing, Queen Elizabeth the Queen Mother Hospital
States of Guernsey, Health and Social Services
States of Jersey, Health and Social Services
Ulster Independent Clinic

The professional organisations that support our work and who constitute our Steering Group:

Association of Anaesthetists of Great Britain and Ireland
Association of Surgeons of Great Britain and Ireland
Coroners' Society of England and Wales
Faculty of Dental Surgery of the Royal College of Surgeons of England
Faculty of Public Health of the Royal College of Physicians of the UK
Institute of Healthcare Management
Royal College of Anaesthetists
Royal College of Child Health and Paediatrics
Royal College of General Practitioners
Royal College of Nursing
Royal College of Obstetricians and Gynaecologists
Royal College of Ophthalmologists
Royal College of Pathologists
Royal College of Physicians of London
Royal College of Radiologists
Royal College of Surgeons of England

The authors and Trustees of NCEPOD would particularly like to thank the NCEPOD staff for their hard work in collecting and analysing the data for this study:

Robert Alleway, Sabah Begg, Philip Brown, Heather Cooper, Karen Protopapa, Sidhaarth Gobin, Clare Holtby, Dolores Jarman, Viki Pepper, and Saba Raza.

In addition we thank our scientific advisors *Dr Martin Utley* and *Professor Steve Gallivan* for all their assistance.

DISCLAIMER

This work was undertaken by NCEPOD, which received funding for this report from the National Patient Safety Agency. The views expressed in this publication are those of the authors and not necessarily those of the Agency.

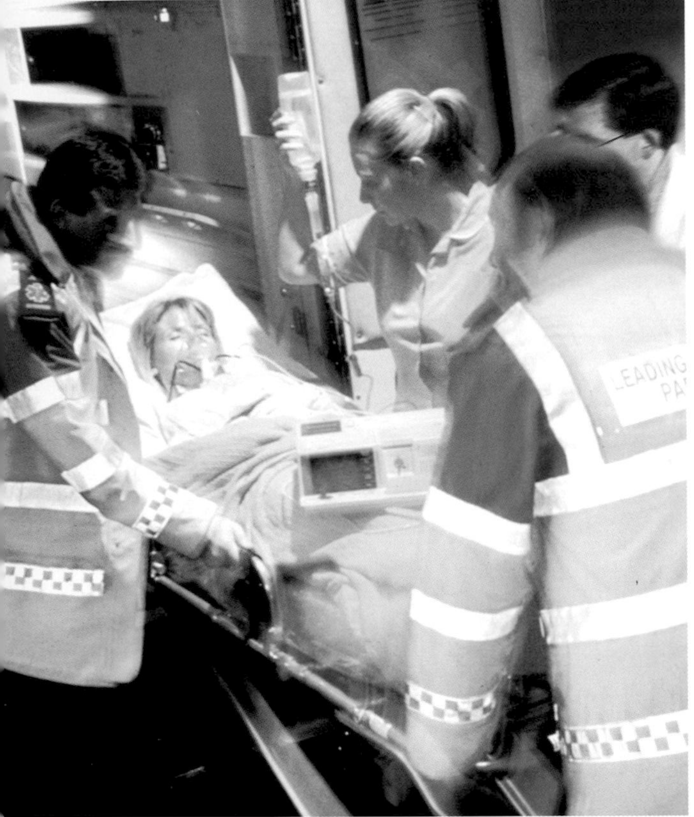

Foreword

Severe injury - a car crash, a fall from a height - accidents such as these are the commonest causes of loss of life in the young. The chance of survival and the completeness of recovery are highly dependent on the care that follows. Some are killed outright but those who survive the initial impact may still die in the hours, days or weeks that follow. The speed with which lethal processes are identified and halted makes the difference between life and death. The injury sets in train life threatening effects of injury on the circulation, tissue oxygenation and the brain. The sooner we can halt and reverse these processes, the more likely and complete will be the return to health.

As a junior in the emergency and neurosurgical departments in Cambridge in the early 1970s we were trained in these rather obvious principles. To use a current catch phrase - it's not rocket science or another, nearer the point - it doesn't take a brain surgeon to work that out! And yet somehow the apparently obvious - or we might see it as "common sense" - was not so commonplace. Then in 1976 an orthopaedic surgeon James Styner crashed his plane in Nebraska. His wife was dead and there he was in a field with three of his four children critically injured. He flagged down a car to get to the nearest hospital - which was closed. Once opened it became clear to him that the care available was inadequate and inappropriate.

The minutes and first hours after an accident are not the time to be working out care from first principles. We miss the obvious under pressure; we cannot hope to make consistently inspired diagnoses. It is not the time to be negotiating a hierarchy, debating priorities and searching shelves and drawers for equipment. We need a well worked out process based on getting most things right and very few things wrong. Realising this, Styner started to work out a system of care. From his initial efforts came Acute Trauma Life Support (ATLS) and with it a new philosophy of care of the severely injured patient based around well thought through processes and teams trained in them - all adhering to the same workshop manual.

To be effective, all processes, including ATLS and other components of care of severely injured patients, must be embedded in practice at every stage: the scene of the accident; alerts to the hospital; the journey from the scene to the emergency department; preparations made there; expertise accessible on arrival and at all subsequent stages, including transfer to specialist services. This NCEPOD report has studied how well we do - and where we sometimes fail. It is by sympathetically, and analytically, studying where things go wrong that we can learn most.

Professor T. Treasure
Chairman

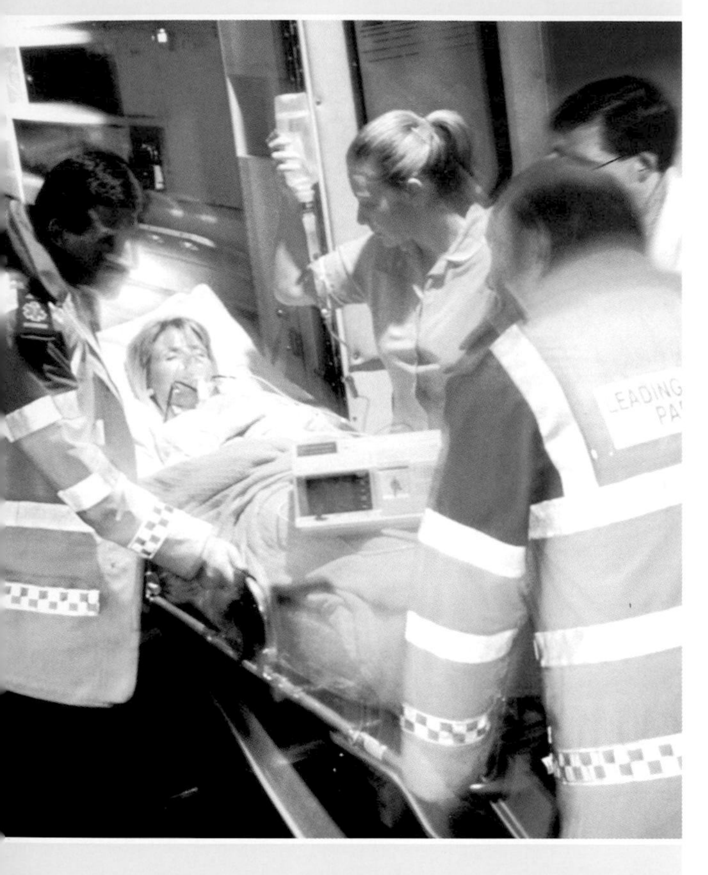

Summary of findings

This study shows a rounded picture of current trauma care provision in England, Wales, Northern Ireland and the Offshore Islands. It draws on data provided by the clinicians involved in the care of these patients (from questionnaires) and data extracted from the casenotes. However, these data are accompanied by peer review, by practising clinicians involved in the day-to-day care of trauma patients, to give a much richer picture than a purely quantitative assessment would allow.

Almost 60% of the patients in this study received a standard of care that was less than good practice. Deficiencies in both organisational and clinical aspects of care occurred frequently.

There were difficulties in identifying those patients with an injury severity score (ISS) >16. With large costs involved in both the provision of care and resources for the management of these patients it is surprising that that there is no current method of identifying the demand for the management of these patients.

The organisation of prehospital care, the trauma team response, seniority of staff involvement and immediate in-hospital care was found to be deficient in many cases.

Lack of appreciation of severity of illness, of urgency of clinical scenario and incorrect clinical decision making were apparent. Many of these clinical issues were related to the lack of seniority and experience of the staff involved in the immediate management of these patients.

It was clear that the provision of suitably experienced staff during evenings and nights was much lower than at other times. In the management of trauma, which very often presents at night, this is a major concern. NHS Trusts should be open about the differences in care by day and night and look to address this as a matter of urgency. Public awareness of these differences may be useful in any debate about the future configuration of trauma services.

Severe trauma is not common and many hospitals see less than one severely injured patient per week. This has a direct bearing on experience and ability to manage these challenging patients. Not only does this relate to clinical skills but also to the feasibility of providing the entire infrastructure required to manage the trauma patient definitively in all centres.

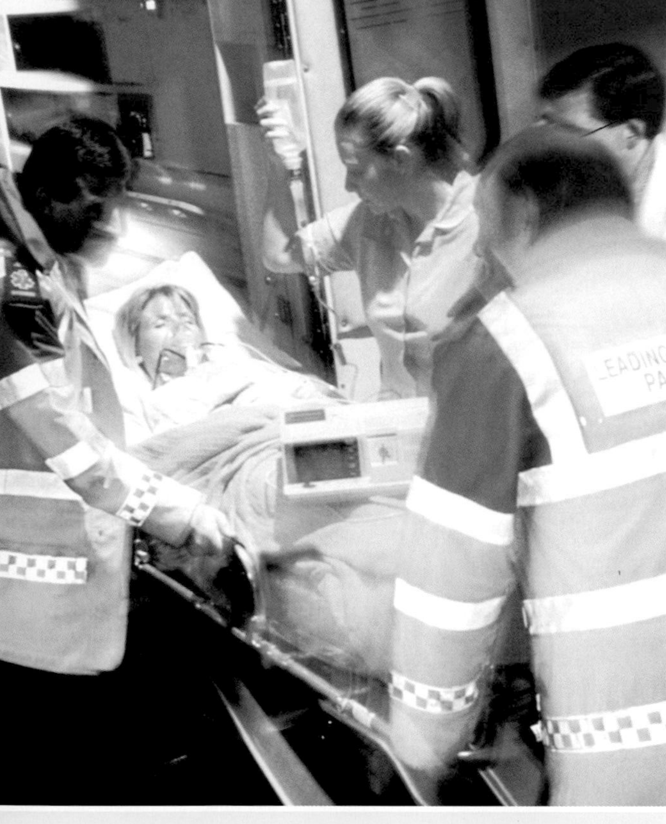

Principal recommendations

Organisational data

There is a need for designated Level 1 trauma centres and a verification process needs to be developed to quality assure the delivery of trauma care (as has been developed in the USA by the American College of Surgeons). *(Royal College of Surgeons of England, College of Emergency Medicine)*

Prehospital care

All agencies involved in trauma management, including emergency medical services, should be integrated into the clinical governance programmes of a regional trauma service. *(All healthcare providers)*

Airway management in trauma patients is often challenging. The prehospital response for these patients should include someone with the skill to secure the airway, (including the use of rapid sequence intubation), and maintain adequate ventilation. *(Ambulance and hospital trusts)*

Hospital reception

Trusts should ensure that a trauma team is available 24 hours a day, seven days a week. This is an essential part of an organised trauma response system. *(Hospital trusts)*

A consultant must be the team leader for the management of the severely injured patient. There should be no reason for this not to happen during the normal working week. Trusts and consultants should work together to provide job plans that will lead to better consultant presence in the emergency department at all times to provide more uniform consultant leadership for all severely injured patients. *(Hospital trusts and clinical directors)*

Airway and breathing

The current structure of prehospital management is insufficient to meet the needs of the severely injured patient. There is a high incidence of failed intubation and a high incidence of patients arriving at hospital with a partially or completely obstructed airway. Change is urgently required to provide a system that reliably provides a clear airway with good oxygenation and control of ventilation. This may be through the provision of personnel with the ability to provide anaesthesia and intubation in the prehospital phase or the use of alternative airway devices. *(Ambulance trusts)*

Management of circulation

Trauma laparotomy is potentially extremely challenging and requires consultant presence within the operating theatre. *(Clinical directors)*

If CT scanning is to be performed, all necessary images should be obtained at the same time. Routine use of 'top to toe' scanning is recommended in the adult trauma patient if no indication for immediate intervention exists. *(Royal College of Radiology and radiology department heads)*

Head injury management

Patients with severe head injury should have a CT head scan of the head performed as soon as possible after admission and within one hour of arrival at hospital. *(Trauma team leader and radiology heads)*

All patients with severe head injury should be transferred to a neurosurgical/critical care centre irrespective of the requirement for surgical intervention. *(Strategic health authorities, hospital trusts, trauma team leaders)*

Paediatric care

Each receiving unit should have up to date guidelines for children which recognise the paediatric skills available on site and their limitations and include agreed guidelines for communication and transfer with specialised paediatric services within the local clinical network. *(Strategic health authorities and hospital trusts)*

Transfers

There should be standardised transfer documentation of the patients' details, injuries, results of investigations and management with records kept at the dispatching and receiving hospitals. *(Trauma team leader, Department of Health)*

Published guidelines must be adhered to and audits performed of the transfers and protocols. *(Hospital trusts)*

Incidence of trauma and organistation of trauma services

Given the relatively low incidence of severe trauma in the UK, it is unlikely that each individual hospital can deliver optimum care to this challenging group of patients. Regional planning for the effective delivery of trauma services is therefore essential. *(Strategic health authorities, hospital trusts)*

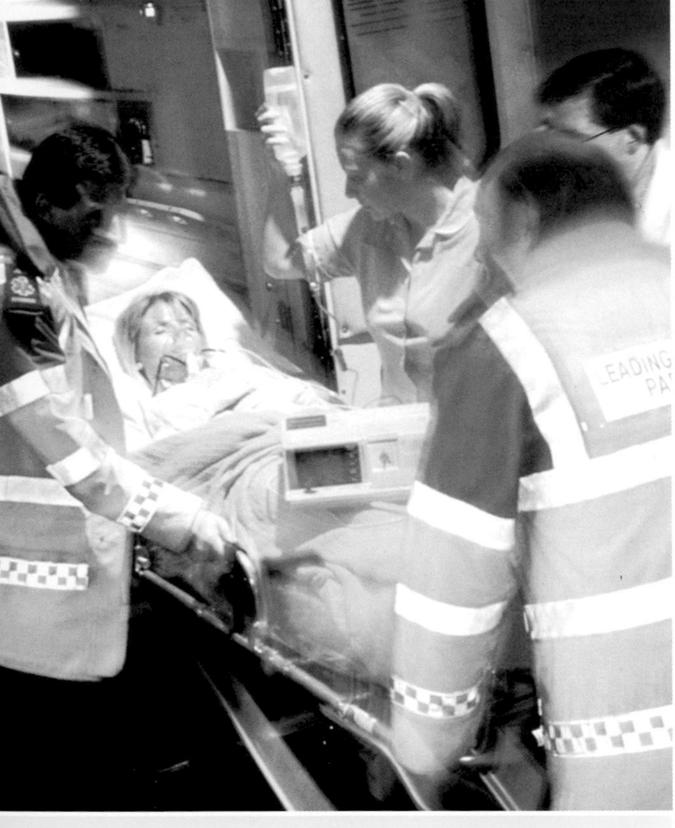

Introduction

Trauma remains the fourth leading cause of death in western countries and the leading cause of death in the first four decades of life. The incidence of trauma is particularly high in the younger population; an average of 36 life years are lost per trauma death[1]. Furthermore, trauma is also a major cause of debilitating long-term injuries. For each trauma fatality there are two survivors with serious or permanent disability[2]. Trauma is, therefore, not only a leading cause of death but also a large socio-economic burden. In 1998, the estimated cost to the NHS, of treating all injuries, was £1.2 billion per annum[3]. Reducing injuries is, therefore, a key government objective. By 2010, the Department of Health aims to have reduced the incidence of accidents by at least 20% from the baseline that was set in 1996[3].

Road trauma accounts for over a third of all deaths due to injury[4]. In 2001-2003, there were (on average) 3,460 traffic related fatalities per annum in Great Britain[5]. The incidence of severe trauma, defined as an Injury Severity Score (ISS) of 16 or greater, is estimated to be four per million per week[6]. Given that the UK population in mid-2003 was in the region of 59.5 million[7], there are approximately 240 severely injured patients in the UK each week.

In 1988, the working party report by the Royal College of Surgeons of England highlighted 'serious deficiencies in the management of severely injured patients'[8]. Following this report, there was increased focus on the care of trauma patients in the UK and consequently the fatality rate of trauma patients reduced. However, most of the improvement in the outcome of these patients occurred prior to 1995, with no further significant change occurring between 1994 and 2000[9].

In 2000, a joint report from the Royal College of Surgeons of England and the British Orthopaedic Association recommended that standards of care for the severely injured patient should be nationally co-ordinated and systematically audited[6]. It was also recommended that standards and outcome measures be developed, against which institutions can audit the outcome of treatment. The standards of care recommended in the report include the use of advance warning systems by the ambulance service, the establishment of trauma teams, the involvement of a senior anaesthetist from the outset and criteria for the activation of the trauma team. The overall purpose of these recommendations was to improve the care of severely injured patients in terms of reduced mortality and unnecessary morbidity.

A number of UK-based single and multi-centre studies have addressed specific issues relating to the care of trauma patients[10-15]. The use of ambulance crews to alert hospitals of severely injured patients, the effect of inter-hospital transfers and the determinants affecting outcome have all been studied. One of the largest UK-based studies looked at the treatment of neurosurgical trauma patients in non-neurosurgical units[16]. There has not, however, been a national study to examine the overall care of trauma patients in the UK to date.

Much of the research on trauma care in the UK has been carried out using data from the Trauma Audit and Research Network (TARN), which was established in response to the Royal College of Surgeons of England's working party report. Approximately 50% of trauma receiving hospitals submit data to TARN[17]. The Trauma Network Database is now an important source of epidemiological data and, in 2000 it contained information on over 120,000 cases[18]. The Healthcare Commission is working with TARN to increase participation from 50% to 100% of hospitals and to expand the number of quantitative trauma audits. At a local level, the feedback provided by TARN to individual hospitals highlights, amongst others, those cases in which patient outcome was 'unexpected'. This markedly aids internal audit and the review of trauma cases by those multi-specialty clinicians who were involved in the care of particular patients. Together with national evaluations of trauma care, in particular head injury, processes of trauma care are also analysed and provide a factual basis for system review.

A lack of continued improvement in outcome is coupled with concern that the quality of care in hospital is not of a consistently high standard across the UK, despite the availability of guidelines that indicate referral pathways for optimum triage, management and access to specialist care[6,19,20]. Furthermore, owing to the incidence of severe trauma, hospitals are unlikely to treat more than one severely injured patient per week. It has been suggested, therefore, that as sufficient trauma experience cannot be achieved at all hospitals, optimal outcomes may be compromised. One of the overall recommendations of the 2000 report was the establishment of a National Trauma Service trauma hub and spoke network between hospitals in each geographic area[6].

The organisation of trauma services in the UK remains highly topical. The recent report from The Royal College of Surgeons of England (2006)[6] confirms that high quality trauma care is not consistently available within the NHS. Recent public debate and government statements reflect the continuing controversies regarding the optimum system of delivering trauma services within the present resource constraints[21]. This study is therefore timely as it explores the organisation in trauma services from the perspective of the patient journey. NCEPOD have identified remediable factors and made recommendations for improvement in the management of the severely injured patient.

The Royal College of Surgeons of England Trauma Committee proposed this study as part of NCEPOD's topic selection process in February 2004. The NCEPOD Steering Group selected the topic, which falls under NCEPOD's extended remit.

References

1. Chaira 0, Cimbanissi S. *Organized trauma care: does volume matter and do trauma centers save lives?* Curr Opin Crit Care 2003; 9:510-4

2. *http://www. tarn.ac.uk/content/images/53/overview% 2006.pdf*

3. *Our Healthier Nation – A contract for Health.* Department of Health, 1998

4. The Royal College of Surgeons of England and the British Orthopaedic Society. *Better Care for the Severely Injured.* 2000

5. Department for Transport, Table 33, *Casualties: by age, road user type and severity: 2001, 2002 and 2003*

6. Gorman DF, Teanby DN, Sinha MP, Wotherspoon J, Boot DA, Molokhia A. *The epidemiology of major injuries in Mersey and North Wales. Injury 1995*; 26(1):51-4

7. Office for National Statistics *http://www.statistics.gov.uk/*

8. *Report of the working party on the management of patients with major injury.* Royal College of Surgeons of England, London. 1988

9. Lecky FE, Woodford M, Bouamra O, Yates DW, on behalf of the Trauma Audit and Research Network. *Lack of change in trauma care in England and Wales since 1994.* Emerg Med J 2002; 19:520-3

10. Crystal R, Bleetman A, Steyn R. *Ambulance crew assessment of trauma severity and alerting practice for trauma patients brought to a general hospital.* Resuscitation 2004; 60:279-82

11. Oakley PA, MacKenzie G, Templeton J, Cook AL, Kirby RM. *Longitudinal trends in trauma mortality and survival in Stoke-on-Trent 1992-1998.* Injury 2004; 35:379-85

12. McGinn GH, MacKenzie RE, Donnelly JA, Smith EA, Runcie CJ. *Interhospital transfer of the critically ill trauma patient: the potential role of a specialist transport system.* J Accid Emerg Med 1996; 13:90-2

13. Cooke RS, McNicholl BP, Byrnes DP. *Early management of severe head injury in Northern Ireland.* Injury 1995; 26(6):395-7

14. Lloyd DA, Patterson M, Robson J, Phillips B. *A stratified response system for the emergency management of the severely injured.* Ann R Coll Surg Engl 2001; 83:15-20

15. Clayton TJ, Nelson RJ, Manara AR. *Reduction in mortality from severe head injury following introduction of a protocol for intensive care management.* British Journal of Anaesthesia 2004; 93(6):761-7

16. McKeating EG, Andrews PJD, Tocher JI, Menon DK. *The intensive care of severe head injury: a survey of non-neurosurgical centres in the United Kingdom.* British Journal of Neurosurgery 1998; 12(1):7-14

17. Lecky F, Woodford M, Yates DW. *Trends in trauma care in England and Wales 1989-1997.* Lancet 2000; 355:1771-5

18. The First Decade 1990-2000. Trauma Audit and Research Network, 2000

19. Report of the Working Party on the Management of Patients with Head Injuries. Royal College of Surgeons of England, London. 1999

20. Triage, assessment, investigation and early management of head injury in infants, children and adults: NICE guidelines, 2003

21. Darzi A. Framework for Action. 2007. *http://www.healthcareforlondon.nhs.uk/framework _for_action.asp*

Method

Study aim

The aim of this study was to examine the process of care for severely injured patients and identify variations that affect the achievement of agreed endpoints.

The expert group identified six main thematic areas that would address the overall aim of the study:

1. Timeliness of events making up the clinical management process.

2. Issues associated with prehospital care at the site of injury and transfer to hospital.

3. Issues associated with the care team that performs the initial resuscitation.

4. Processes and procedures associated with secondary transfers.

5. Issues associated with pathways, handovers and communication.

6. Membership of the Trauma Audit Research Network (TARN).

Expert group

A multidisciplinary group of experts comprising clinicians from emergency medicine, general surgery, neurosurgery, radiology, anaesthetics, and lay representatives contributed to the design of the study and reviewed the combined analysis of the data; both from the questionnaires and the extra information from the advisory groups.

Case identification

Patients were identified prospectively. A nominated contact in the emergency department identified patients as severely injured based primarily on their, and their colleagues', clinical judgement. A list of patients (which included a patient identifier and the date and time of admission) was then forwarded to the NCEPOD local reporter who completed a monthly spreadsheet which contained additional information (for example, the name of the admitting clinician). Data collection ran for three months from February 1st 2006 to April 30th 2006. Patients of all ages were eligible for inclusion. After each month of sampling, a spreadsheet was returned, password-protected, to NCEPOD along with photocopies of all of the casenotes for the first 72 hours in hospital. The casenotes were used by NCEPOD staff to calculate an injury severity score (ISS) for each patient (see Appendix B). Patients with an ISS of 16 or more were included in the study. The casenotes of included patients were subsequently used for the peer review process.

Exclusions

The following patient groups were excluded:

Death by hanging or drowning (the pathology is asphyxia rather than trauma); and

Patients brought in for confirmation of death.

Questionnaires and casenotes

There were three questionnaires used to collect data for this study, two clinical questionnaires per patient and one organisational questionnaire per site.

1. A&E clinician questionnaire
This questionnaire was sent to the A&E clinician in charge of the patient's initial resuscitation. Information was requested concerning the mode and time of arrival, initial trauma response, timeliness of investigations and hospital transfers.

2. Admitting consultant questionnaire
This questionnaire concerned information on the location and consultant specialty to which the patient was admitted. It also contained information on surgical procedures, patient outcome and secondary transfers.

3. Organisational questionnaire
This questionnaire concerned data on the staff, departments, facilities and protocols for each participating hospital. Information was collected at the hospital level as it gave a better indication of the facilities available for a patient at the location where they were receiving care, rather than all the facilities available within the trust as a whole.

The organisational questionnaire was sent to the medical director for completion. If, after a reminder, it was not returned to NCEPOD a copy was sent to the NCEPOD local reporter of that hospital. Clinical questionnaires were either sent to the NCEPOD local reporter for dissemination or directly to the clinician involved, depending on the choice of the hospital local reporter. However, whichever method was used, it was requested that the completed questionnaires were returned directly to NCEPOD.

It had been hoped at the outset of the study that, in addition to these questionnaires, some information not otherwise available regarding the prehospital management of patients could be obtained from a questionnaire completed by ambulance crews. However, it proved difficult to agree this with ambulance services, partly due to employment contract issues and partly due to reorganisation of ambulance trusts. Therefore, assessment of prehospital care has been acquired from:

a) The patient report form (PRF); completed by ambulance crews at the scene and en route, a copy of which should be available in the medical records.

b) Advisors' assessments of the prehospital care following review of both the PRF and clinical records and questionnaires completed by the clinicians relating to hospital management.

To complement the data available from the above questionnaires, copies of all the casenotes for patients' first 72 hours in hospital were requested. If the patient was transferred within 72 hours, the casenotes from the receiving hospital were also requested.

Advisor group

A multidisciplinary group of advisors was recruited to review the casenotes and associated questionnaires. The group of advisors comprised clinicians from the following specialties: emergency medicine, anaesthetics, general surgery, intensive care medicine, maxillofacial surgery, neurosurgery, nursing, paediatrics, plastics, orthopaedics and vascular surgery.

For each case reviewed, the advisor completed an assessment form. This allowed both quantitative and qualitative analysis of the advisor's opinion.

Specific sections of the assessment form were completed by NCEPOD researchers using information extracted from the casenotes such as the times of investigations, Airway, Breathing, Circulation (ABC) measurements and the grades of doctors involved in the patients' care. The remainder of the assessment form was completed by the advisors who were asked to provide expert opinion on the prehospital care, trauma response, timeliness of investigations and the overall care of the patient.

Peer review process

All questionnaires and casenotes were anonymised by the non-clinical staff at NCEPOD. All patient, clinician and hospital identifiers were removed. Neither clinical staff at NCEPOD, nor the advisors had access to any identifiable information.

After being anonymised each case was reviewed by one advisor within a multidisciplinary group. At regular intervals throughout the meeting, the chair allowed a period of discussion for each advisor to summarise their cases and ask for opinions from other specialties or raise aspects of a case for discussion.

The grading system below was used by the advisors to grade the overall care each patient received.

Good practice:
A standard that you would accept from yourself, your trainees and your institution.

Room for improvement:
Aspects of **clinical** care that could have been better.

Room for improvement:
Aspects of **organisational** care that could have been better.

Room for improvement:
Aspects of **both clinical** and **organisational** care that could have been better.

Less than satisfactory:
Several aspects of **clinical** and/or **organisational** care that were well below that you would accept from yourself, your trainees and your institution.

Insufficient information submitted to assess the quality of care.

Quality and confidentiality

A number of predetermined, mandatory key fields on each questionnaire had been set to ensure that data analysis could be performed effectively. If these key fields were not completed on receipt of the questionnaire by NCEPOD, the NCEPOD local reporter or clinician was contacted to see if the data could be obtained.

Each case was given a unique NCEPOD number so that cases could not easily be linked to a hospital.

The data from all questionnaires received were electronically scanned into a preset database. Prior to any analysis taking place, the data were cleaned to ensure that there were no duplicate records and that erroneous data had not been entered during scanning. Any fields that contained spurious data that could not be validated were removed.

Data analysis

Following cleaning of the quantitative data, descriptive statistics were produced.

The qualitative data collected from the assessment form and free text answers in the clinical questionnaires were coded according to content and context. The data were reviewed by NCEPOD clinical staff to identify the nature and frequency of recurring themes.

Case studies have been used throughout this report to illustrate particular themes.

All data were analysed using Microsoft Access and Excel by the staff at NCEPOD.

The findings of the report were reviewed by the expert group, advisors and the NCEPOD steering group prior to publication.

CHAPTER 1 - Data overview

Hospital participation

An organisational questionnaire was completed for 183/218 (83.9%) hospitals, that were expected to participate.

Patient identifier spreadsheets

A patient identifier spreadsheet was returned for 180/218 (82.6%) hospitals that were expected to participate. In total this equated to 2203 patients, for which NCEPOD received 1735 (78.8%) sets of casenotes to calculate an injury severity score (ISS). Of these 909 cases had an ISS less than 16 and 826 patients had an ISS ≥ 16, 31 of which were excluded as they were either dead on arrival, had complications of a previous injury or there was insufficient information for the advisors to assess any aspect of the patient's care. The remaining 795 patients were included in the study sample.

Clinician questionnaires

The study was designed such that the overwhelming majority of the quantitative and qualitative data could be obtained directly from the casenotes and the focussed opinions of the advisors' (i.e. from the advisor assessment form). To supplement this, the clinician responsible for the initial resuscitation of the patient and the admitting consultant (if applicable) were asked to complete a patient care questionnaire. In total 513 A&E clinician questionnaires and 432 admitting consultant questionnaires were returned.

Age and gender

Seventy five percent (594/795) of the patients were males, and the mean age of the whole sample was 39.6 years. The mode age of the study sample was 18; one in six (128/795) patients being 16 – 20 years old (Figure 1).

Figure 1. Age range of patient sample

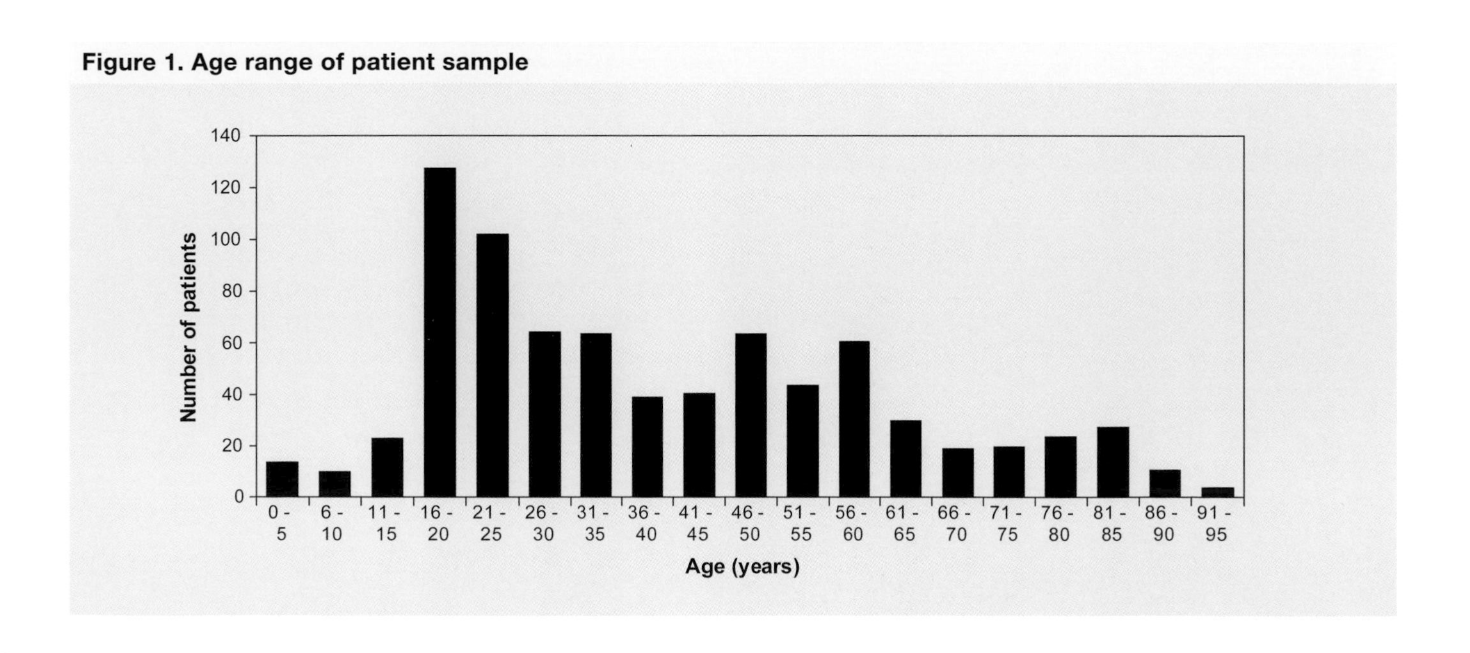

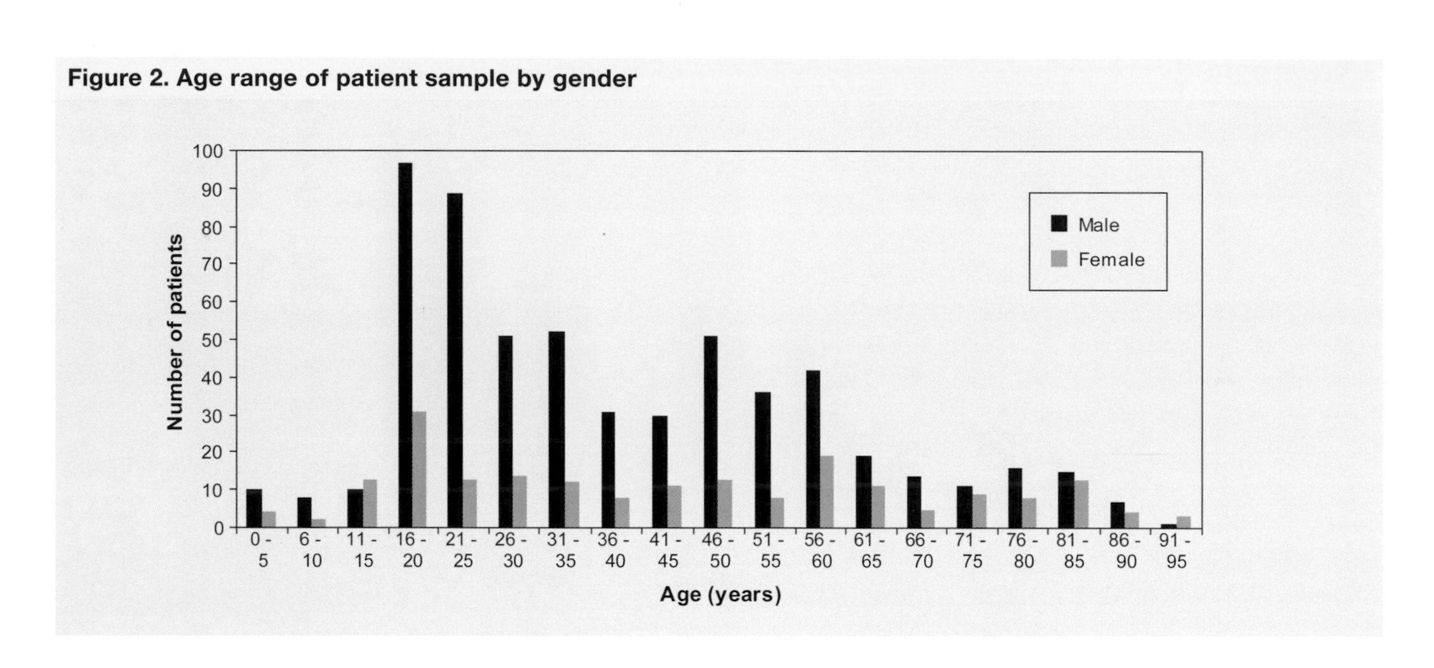

Figure 2. Age range of patient sample by gender

Figure 2 shows the age range analysed by gender. The mean age for males was 38 and mean age for females 44. There was a peak in frequency for males aged 16-25.

Of the patients in the study 56.3% (442/785) were involved in a road traffic collision (RTC) (Table 1).

Table 1. Mechanism of injury

	Number of patients	%
RTC (driver/passenger)	319	40.6
RTC (pedestrian)	123	15.7
Fall from height	136	17.3
Assault	72	9.2
Industrial/agricultural	21	2.7
Sport/leisure	18	2.3
Self harm	15	1.9
Other	81	10.3
Subtotal	**785**	
Not recorded	10	
Total	**795**	

Day and time of arrival

The number of severely injured patients presenting to the emergency department peaked on Friday and Saturday (Figure 3).

The rise in number of patients on Friday and Saturday was largely due to an increase in patients arriving at night ('out of hours') at the weekend (see Table 2). Daytime admissions were largely constant and were actually lower than the weekly average on Friday and Saturday. The mean age of the patients who presented out of hours on Friday, Saturday and Sunday was considerably lower than the remainder of the population: 33.5 years compared to 42.3 years.

Figure 3. Patient arrivals by day of week

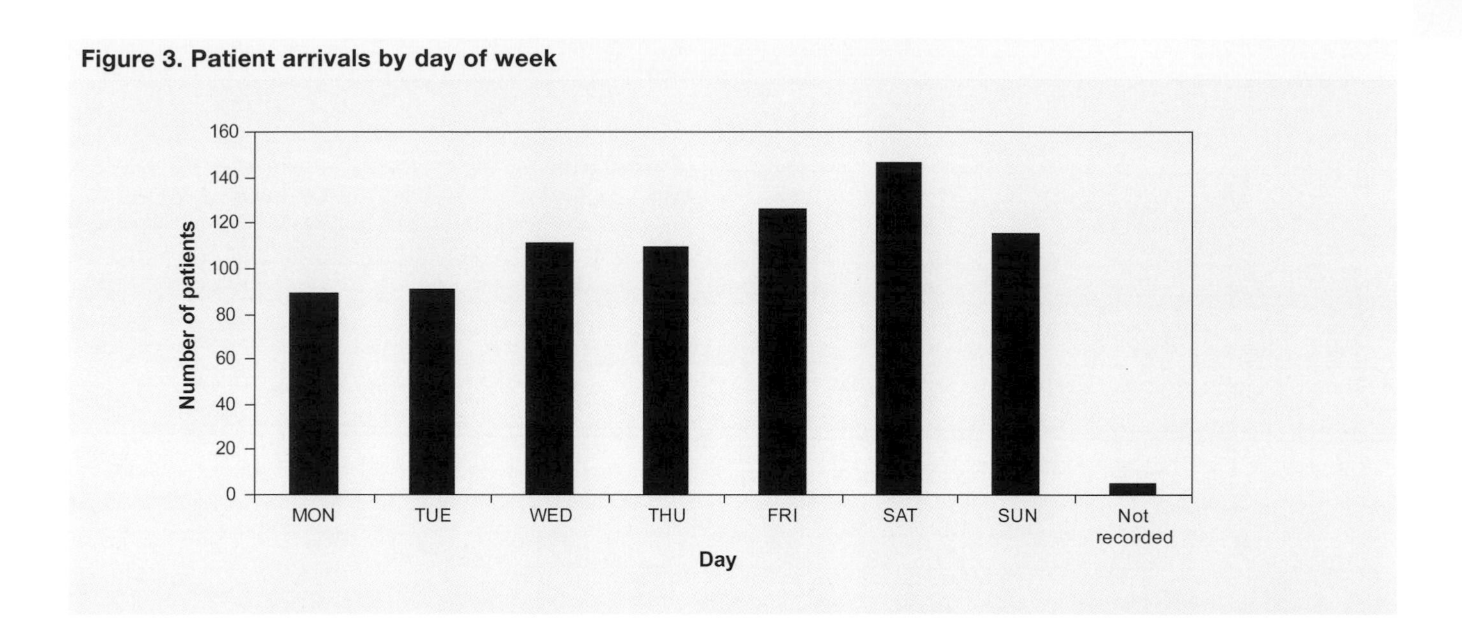

Table 2. Patient arrivals by time of day and day of week

	Day 08.00-17.59		Night 18.00-07.59				
		%		%	Subtotal	Time of day not recorded	Total
Mon	41	47.1	46	52.9	**87**	2	**89**
Tue	56	63.6	32	36.4	**88**	3	**91**
Wed	59	53.6	51	46.4	**110**	1	**111**
Thu	54	49.1	56	50.9	**110**	0	**110**
Fri	50	44.6	72	59.0	**122**	4	**126**
Sat	46	32.2	97	67.8	**143**	4	**147**
Sun	38	36.9	65	63.1	**103**	13	**116**
Subtotal	**344**		**419**		**763**	**27**	**790**
Day not recorded	0		0		**0**	5	**5**
Total	**344**		**419**		**763**	**32**	**795**

Mode of arrival

Table 3. Mode of arrival to hospital

	Number of patients	%
Ambulance	652	83.3
Helicopter	92	11.7
Other emergency service	5	<1
Hospital transfer	9	1.1
Member of public	13	1.7
Self referral	8	1.0
Other	4	<1
Subtotal	**783**	
Not recorded	12	
Total	**795**	

The majority of patients 652/783 (83.3%) were transported to hospital by road ambulance. A further 92/783 (11.7%) patients arrived by helicopter. Only 25 patients arrived by means other than an emergency service vehicle (Table 3).

Injury severity scores

Table 4. Injury severity score

	Number of patients	%
16 – 24	449	56.5
25 – 35	279	35.1
36 – 75	67	8.4
Total	**795**	

Table 4 summarises the ISS of the study patient population.

Table 5. Patient outcome at 72 hours by ISS

ISS	Alive	Deceased	Total	% Mortality
16 – 24	411	38	**449**	8.5
25 – 35	220	59	**269**	21.9
36 – 75	47	20	**67**	29.9
Total	**678**	**117**	**795**	**14.7**

The 72 hour outcome for each ISS group is shown in Table 5.

There was an increased mortality with increased injury severity.

Table 6. Injuries by body region (answers may be multiple)

	Number of patients
Head	493
Face	191
Neck	14
Thorax	388
Abdomen and pelvic contents	143
Spine	162
Upper extremity	224
Lower extremity	289
External	82

Table 6 summarises the injuries by body region.

CHAPTER 2 - Organisational data

This chapter summarises the collated data from the 183 hospitals that returned a completed organisational questionnaire. It provides the reader with an overview of the departments, facilities, staff and protocols that were available for the care of severely injured patients during the study period.

Departments and procedures

Table 7 summarises the departments and/or procedures that were available at the participating hospitals. It should be noted that some hospitals without a specific department e.g. vascular surgery, did have staff that were able to perform surgical procedures related to that specialty.

The most striking, albeit well known fact, was the small number of hospitals that had a neurosurgery department (31) or performed neurosurgical procedures (a further seven hospitals). This is of particular concern given the large number of severely injured patients who suffered neurotrauma as part of their constellation of injuries (over 60% of patients in this study). The availability in patient services is also reflected in the Transfer chapter later in this report. By far the most common reason for a secondary transfer was the requirement for neurosurgery and/or neurological monitoring. Time to definitive neurosurgical intervention can be a major determinant of outcome for patients with traumatic brain injury and the requirement for a secondary transfer to access neurosurgical services lengthens this time (see Time to surgery page 106).

More than half of the patients in the current study presented to the emergency department out of hours. Furthermore, many required immediate treatment. While in the large majority of hospitals procedures were available for orthopaedic trauma (168/173) and general surgery (166/173) out of hours, immediate intervention for more specialised injuries was often not available.

Table 7. Overview of departments and procedures

	Department on site	Department not on site but specialty procedures available		Subtotal	Not answered	Total
	Yes	Yes	No			
Orthopaedic trauma	166	7	9	**182**	1	**183**
Neurosurgery	31	7	132	**170**	13	**183**
General surgery	173	2	7	**182**	1	**183**
Vascular surgery	131	15	33	**179**	4	**183**
Plastic surgery	44	30	98	**172**	11	**183**
Cardiac surgery	28	7	136	**171**	12	**183**
Thoracic surgery	31	24	115	**170**	13	**183**
Maxillofacial surgery	111	13	53	**177**	6	**183**
ENT	137	14	28	**179**	4	**183**
Urology	153	13	15	**181**	2	**183**
Vascular interventional radiology	108	19	47	**174**	9	**183**

Table 8. Availability of multiple 24 hour treatment

Emergency department	Emergency department	Emergency department	Emergency department	Emergency department	Emergency department	Emergency department
	General surgery	General surgery	General surgery	General surgery	General surgery	General surgery
		Orthopaedic trauma	Orthopaedic trauma	Orthopaedic trauma	Orthopaedic trauma	Orthopaedic trauma
			Vascular surgery	Vascular surgery	Vascular surgery	Vascular surgery
				Neurosurgery	Cardiac or Thoracic surgery	Neurosurgery
						Cardiac or Thoracic surgery
183	**166**	**159**	**90**	**23**	**33**	**17**

Table 9. X-ray with immediate reporting by proximity to emergency department and 24 hour accessibility

	24 hour accessibility				
Proximity	**Yes**	**No**	**Subtotal**	**Not answered**	**Total**
Adjacent	112	25	**137**	9	**146**
Onsite not adjacent	15	7	**22**	1	**23**
Offsite	0	2	**2**	0	**2**
Subtotal	**127**	**34**	**161**	**10**	**171**
Not answered	2	4	**6**	6	**12**
Total	**129**	**38**	**167**	**16**	**183**

The availability of multiple specialty treatment was further analysed. It is clear from Table 8 that regional planning of trauma services should consider the availability of services at each hospital and consider whether it is appropriate to take some severely injured patients to hospitals without a full range of services, available at all times. Only 17 hospitals that participated in this study could have been considered for Level 1 verification as a Trauma Centre (see Appendix E).

Twenty four hour accessibility was defined as a facility which can be fully staffed and functional when required anytime of day or night. Thirty four hospitals reported that they did not have x-ray with immediate reporting meeting this definition (Table 9). Such a fundamental facility should be available at all times at every hospital that has the potential to receive a severely injured patient.

Whilst 161/169 (95.3%) hospitals had CT scanning that met the 24 hour definition, only 97/169 (57.4%) had the scanners located adjacent to the emergency department

Table 10. CT scanner and access to immediate reporting; proximity to emergency department and 24 hour accessibility

	24 hour accessibility				
Proximity	**Yes**	**No**	**Subtotal**	**Not answered**	**Total**
Adjacent	93	4	**97**	6	**103**
Onsite not adjacent	68	4	**72**	4	**76**
Subtotal	**161**	**8**	**169**	**10**	**179**
Not answered	2	0	**2**	2	**4**
Total	**163**	**8**	**171**	**12**	**183**

(Table 10). Since the risk to a patient's stability is increased during movement, close proximity of the CT scanner to the patient in the emergency department is of huge importance. It should be noted that advisors and clinicians completing questionnaires frequently indicated that a patient could not be scanned because of their instability. It is likely that this scenario could be improved by the relocation of CT scanners into the resuscitation room.

In accordance with The Royal College of Radiologists' technical standards for CT[1] there appears to have been a fairly good investment in CT scanner technology, as 117/145 (80.7%) hospitals that answered the question reported having a scanner less than six years old (Table 11). The remaining 28 hospitals should consider updating their CT scanner in line with newer technology.

Table 12 demonstrates excellent access to a blood bank from emergency departments.

Table 11. Age of CT scanners (years)

	Number of hospitals	%
0	11	7.6
1	28	19.3
2	21	14.5
3	13	9.0
4	21	14.5
5	23	15.9
6	10	6.9
7	8	5.5
8	3	2.1
9	5	4.9
10	2	1.4
Subtotal	**145**	
Not answered	38	
Total	**183**	

Table 12. Blood bank location and 24 hour accessibility

	24 hour accessibility				
Proximity	**Yes**	**No**	**Subtotal**	**Not answered**	**Total**
Adjacent	19	0	**19**	3	**22**
Onsite not adjacent	145	0	**145**	10	**155**
Offsite	2	0	**2**	1	**3**
Subtotal	**166**	**0**	**166**	**14**	**180**
Not answered	0	0	**0**	3	**3**
Total	**166**	**0**	**166**	**17**	**183**

Table 13. 24 hour access to haematology and biochemistry investigations

	Haematology	Biochemistry
Yes	165	165
No	1	0
Subtotal	**166**	**165**
Not answered	17	18
Total	**183**	**183**

Table 14. Number of resuscitation bays

	Number of hospitals	%
1	5	2.7
2	19	10.4
3	46	25.3
4	60	33.0
5	29	15.9
6	18	9.9
> 6	5	2.7
Subtotal	**182**	
Not answered	1	
Total	**183**	

Only one hospital was reported not to have access to 24 hour haematology investigations, however a further 17 sites failed to answer the question (Table 13). This finding was similar for the 24 hour accessibility to biochemistry.

The resuscitation bay provides an area and an array of equipment that are essential for the immediate treatment of patients. Since there are often two or more victims from one road traffic collision (RTC), and other seriously ill patients also need to be treated in this location, it is important to note that 70 hospitals had less than four resuscitation bays (Table 14).

Table 15. Equipment available to each resuscitation bay

	Number of hospitals
Anaesthetic machine/head	136
Difficult intubation trolley	149
Positive pressure ventilator	166
SpO_2 monitoring	182
$FeCO_2$ monitoring	158
Central venous pressure monitoring	171
Arterial pressure monitoring	170
Surgical set	146
Cricothyroidotomy set	178
Intercostal drain set	180
Tracheosotomy set	165
Diagnostic peritoneal lavage	144
Cut down set	177
External pelvic fixation set	48
Foley catheter	182
Nasogastric tube	183
Obstetric wedge	87
Rapid infusion equipment	147
Fluid warming equipment	171
Rhesus negative blood	112
Defibrillator	181
Focused Assessment with Sonography for Trauma	61
Portable x-ray	165
Fixed gantry x-ray	56
Portable or fixed gantry x-ray	183

There are some notable findings in Table 15. Many severely injured patients require anaesthesia and tracheal intubation. If already intubated in the prehospital phase, maintenance of anaesthesia will often be required. Despite this, one in four hospitals reported that they did not have anaesthetic machines in each bay and one in ten reported that they did not have ventilators. Rapid investigation of possible intraperitoneal haemorrhage is another essential component in the care of these patients. However, Focussed Assessment with Sonography for Trauma (FAST) was only available in 33.3% (61/183) of emergency departments and diagnostic peritoneal lavage in 78.7% (144/183).

In the 1993/1994 NCEPOD report, it was recommended that all acute hospitals should have a theatre that is kept free from elective surgery in the event that a patient requires an emergency procedure. Such emergency daytime theatres are often referred to as 'NCEPOD theatres'. Table 16 shows that 151/177 (85.3%) hospitals had a NCEPOD theatre, a significant improvement on 1993/1994.

Table 16. Number of hospitals with dedicated emergency and trauma theatres

	Dedicated trauma theatre				
NCEPOD theatre	Yes	No	**Subtotal**	Not answered	**Total**
Yes	129	22	**151**	3	**154**
No	10	16	**26**	1	**27**
Subtotal	**139**	**38**	**177**	**4**	**181**
Not answered	0	1	**1**	1	**2**
Total	**139**	**39**	**178**	**5**	**183**

Table 17. Number of consultants (whole time equivalents) by specialty

	Emergency medicine	Orthopaedic surgeons	General surgeons	Vascular surgeons	Interventional radiologists
0	3	6	2	43	51
> 0 < 1	1	1	0	25	14
≥ 1 < 2	16	2	3	43	32
≥ 2 < 3	29	5	11	29	36
≥ 3 < 4	47	7	16	24	21
≥ 4 < 5	40	21	17	8	6
≥ 5 < 6	21	30	31	1	8
≥ 6	25	101	93	2	6
Subtotal	**182**	**173**	**173**	**175**	**174**
Not answered	1	10	10	8	9
Total	**183**	**183**	**183**	**183**	**183**

Table 18. Number of consultants (whole time equivalents) that took part in the emergency rota

	Orthopaedic surgeons	General surgeons	Vascular surgeons	Interventional radiologists
0	9	12	51	84
> 0 < 1	2	0	18	2
≥ 1 < 2	0	2	35	17
≥ 2 < 3	5	12	23	22
≥ 3 < 4	6	17	19	14
≥ 4 < 5	25	18	6	7
≥ 5 < 6	32	32	2	7
≥ 6	89	78	1	4
Subtotal	**168**	**171**	**155**	**157**
Not answered	15	12	28	26
Total	**183**	**183**	**183**	**183**

Table 19. Number of consultants who had taught on an Advanced Trauma Life Support (ATLS) course in the last two years

	Emergency medicine	Orthopaedic surgeons	General surgeons	Vascular surgeons
0	33	88	119	127
1	43	32	22	13
2	37	21	14	2
3	31	8	3	2
4	11	1	1	1
5	8	3	1	0
≥ 6	11	1	0	0
Subtotal	**174**	**154**	**160**	**145**
Not answered	9	29	23	38
Total	**183**	**183**	**183**	**183**

Table 19 demonstrates that ATLS, at the instructor level, was very much more supported by emergency medicine than surgery – this is in contrast to the USA where surgeons are in charge of the trauma system and trauma education.

Table 20. Number of consultants who had a specialist interest in trauma

	Orthopaedic surgeons	General surgeons	Vascular surgeons	Interventional vascular radiologists
0	66	137	128	123
1	25	10	13	12
2	9	5	6	10
3	9	5	2	4
4	9	1	3	2
5	7	3	0	0
≥ 6	39	6	0	0
Subtotal	**164**	**167**	**152**	**151**
Not answered	19	16	31	32
Total	**183**	**183**	**183**	**183**

The management of trauma patients requires a multidisciplinary approach. However, at the time of this study there was a lack of specialist interest in trauma across the specialties (Table 20). This may well be a reflection of the low trauma workload which makes it difficult to develop and maintain a special interest in this area, given the current configuration of trauma services.

To explore the apparent lack of specific consultant interest in trauma further, we looked at the 33 hospitals that performed neurosurgical procedures at all times. Table 21 demonstrates that even in those hospitals with neurosurgery, other than interest from orthopaedic surgeons there was little specialist interest in trauma. This is important as it has been proposed that hospitals with neurosurgery could form the basis of regional trauma centres[2].

Table 22 illustrates the number of hospitals which had a formal trauma team and whether or not ATLS courses were run onsite. One hundred and forty three hospitals (78.1%) had a formal trauma team, and 82 (44.8%) indicated that they ran ATLS courses onsite. It is difficult to comprehend the finding that 16 hospitals that ran ATLS courses did not have a formal trauma team; a key component of ATLS.

Table 21. Hospitals that perform neurosurgical procedures at all times and consultants with a specialist interest in trauma

	Number of hospitals
Orthopaedic surgeons	24
General surgeons	5
Vascular surgeons	6
Vascular interventional radiologists	5

Table 22. Formal trauma team/response associated with an ATLS course run onsite

	Formal trauma team		
ATLS courses	Yes	No	**Total**
Yes	66	16	**82**
No	77	24	**101**
Total	**143**	**40**	**183**

Table 23. Specialty of trauma team by residency

	Consultant		Emergency Medicine SpR or above		Anaesthetic SpR or above		Surgical SpR or above	
		%		%		%		%
Resident	6	3.3	109	59.6	111	60.7	86	47.0
Non resident	59	32.2	36	19.7	13	7.1	34	18.6
Not present	118	64.5	38	20.8	59	32.2	63	34.4
Total	**183**		**183**		**183**		**183**	

The majority (134/143) of hospitals with a formal trauma team had a written protocol for activating a trauma response.

To determine who would respond to a severely injured patient out of hours, we asked for a list of the grades, specialties, ATLS and residency status, for each of the clinicians who were on call on Sunday February 5th 2006 at 2am.

Despite the recommendation that the trauma team leader should be a consultant[3], the majority of hospitals (118/183) did not have consultant presence for the management of major trauma during the early hours of Sunday morning on February 5th 2006. Furthermore, in only six cases was the consultant a resident and thus immediately available (Table 23).

Immediate airway control is vital. Only 111/183 hospitals (60.7%) had an anaesthetic SpR or above immediately available. Trauma airways are likely to be difficult and an anaesthetic SpR or above should be present immediately in the emergency department.

The management of the severely injured patient can be extremely challenging and rapid, accurate communication of all aspects of care is essential. This is particularly important given that many different specialties may be involved. It can be seen from Table 24 that only 51/175 hospitals had written protocols covering this important area.

Table 24. Communication and handovers

	Written protocol for handing over care			
	Clinical teams		Clinical specialties	
		%		%
Yes	59	33.1	51	29.1
No	119	66.9	124	70.9
Subtotal	**178**		**175**	
Not answered	5		8	
Total	**183**		**183**	

Over a third (65/183) of hospitals indicated that they did not allocate a named person for communicating with the patient/relatives. This insufficiency was reflected by the individual cases. Where the advisors felt they were able to assess the level of communication with the patient/relatives, 31.4% (141/449) of cases were found to be less than satisfactory for quantity and quality of communication. This clearly indicates that a named person of appropriate seniority must be nominated to the patient/relatives as a point of contact. Communication with the patient/relatives must be documented to allow all involved with the care of the patient to be aware of the occurrence and content of this communication.

Key findings

Many severely injured patients are taken to hospitals that do not have the staff or facilities to provide definitive care.

In this study only 17 hospitals had the range of specialities available to be considered for a Level 1 Trauma Centre (under the verification system of the American College of Surgeons).

39.3% (72/183) of hospitals did not have a resident anaesthetist at SpR level or above.

65% (118/183) of hospitals stated that a consultant was not involved in the initial care of a severely injured patient who presented at 0200 on Sunday 5th February 2006.

Recommendations

There is a need for designated Level 1 trauma centres and a verification process needs to be developed to quality assure the delivery of trauma care (as has been developed in USA by the American College of Surgeons). *(Royal College of Surgeons of England, College of Emergency Medicine)*

All hospitals receiving trauma cases should have at least four resuscitation bays. *(Hospital trusts)*

All hospitals receiving trauma patients should have a resident SpR or above with the skills to immediately secure the airway in trauma patients. *(Hospital trusts)*

There should be a CT scanner within or adjacent to the resuscitation room. *(Hospital trusts)*

Each trust involved in trauma care should develop a core group of clinicians with a special interest in trauma management. This trauma care delivery group should include a member of the trust executive staff. *(Hospital trusts)*

References

1. *http://www.rcr.ac.uk/docs/radiology/worddocs/RCRStandardsforCT11thNov2003webed.doc*

2. A Darzi. *Framework for Action*. 2007. *http://www.healthcareforlondon.nhs.uk/framework_for_action.asp*

3. The Royal College of Surgeons of England and the British Orthopaedic Society. *Better Care for the Severely Injured.* 2000

CHAPTER 3 - Overall assessment

All cases

Figure 4 shows the advisors' assessment of overall quality of care for the whole study population. More than half the patients (415/795) were subjected to less than good practice. There was greater room for improvement in organisational (180/795) rather than clinical (129/795) aspects of care.

Overall assessment by volume of cases

Figure 5 shows the overall assessment of care analysed by the volume of cases each hospital reported to NCEPOD during the study period. Hospitals that reported greater than 20 patients during the study period had a higher percentage of cases classed as good practice than centres that reported fewer cases (57% v 39%).

Figure 4. Overall assessment of care (advisors' view)

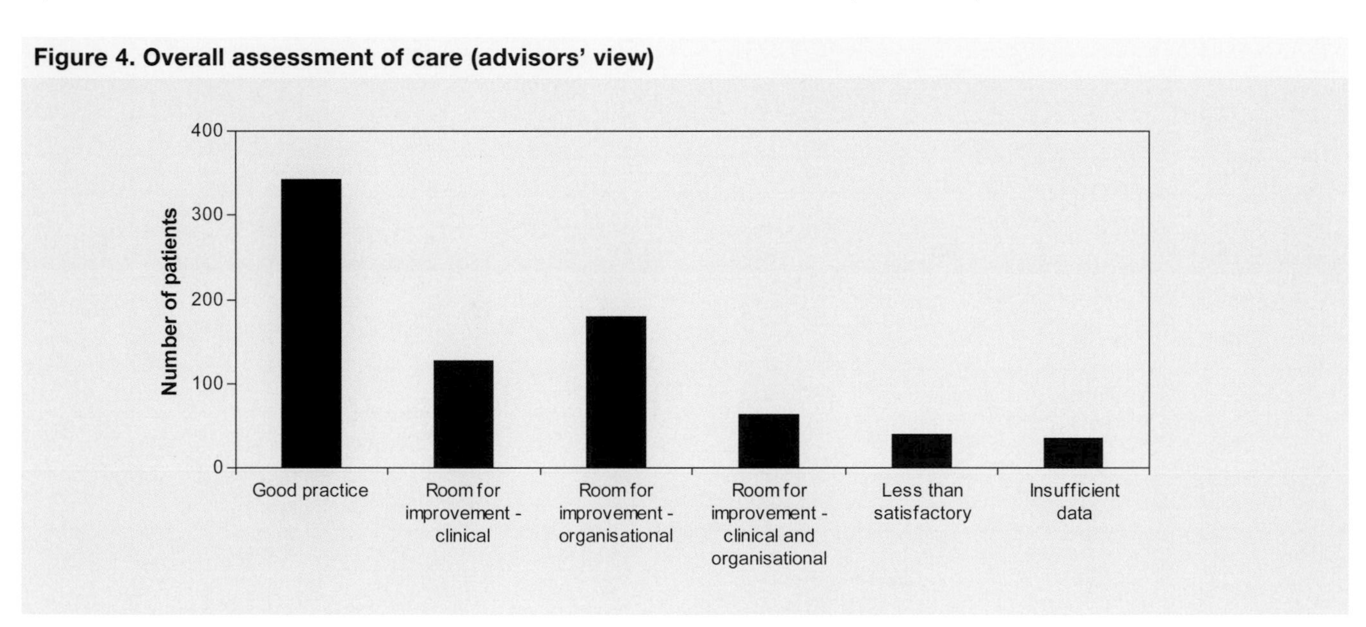

Figure 5. Number of patients per hospital vs. advisors' overall assessment

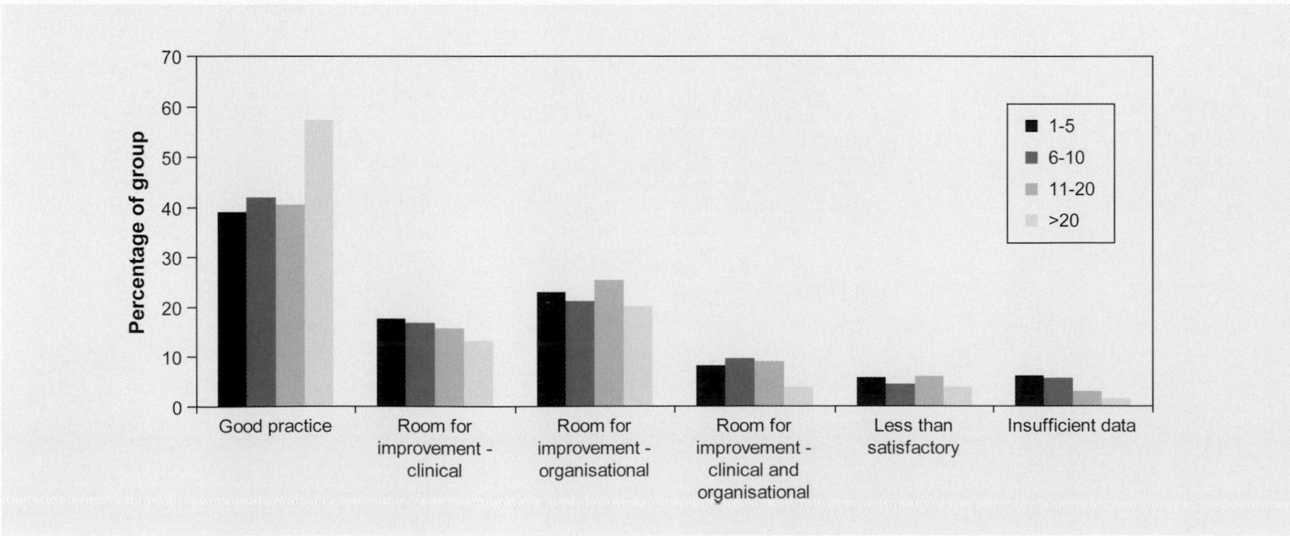

Table 25. Appropriate initial response

	Number of patients	%
Yes	605	86.6
No	94	13.4
Subtotal	**699**	
Insufficient data	96	
Total	**795**	

Table 26. Appropriateness of the response by grade of reviewer

	Appropriate response				
Grade of first reviewer	**Yes**		**No**		**Total**
		%		**%**	
Consultant	154	96.9	5	3.1	**159**
NCCG	16	84.2	3	15.8	**19**
SpR	204	88.3	27	11.7	**231**
SHO	52	76.5	16	23.5	**68**
Total	**426**		**51**		**477**

Table 27. Overall assessment in patients with inappropriate initial response

	Number of patients	%
Good practice	8	8.5
Room for improvement – clinical	28	29.8
Room for improvement – organisational	17	18.1
Room for improvement – clinical and organisational	21	22.3
Less than satisfactory	17	18.1
Insufficient data	3	3.2
Total	**94**	

Appropriateness of initial hospital response

The advisors were asked to assess the initial response to the trauma patient. Table 25 shows that 94/699 (13.4%) cases, where the advisors could make an assessment, were graded as having an inappropriate initial response. In a further 96/795 cases there was insufficient data to comment.

Appropriateness of initial response by grade of staff

Table 26 shows the appropriateness of initial response in cases where the grade of staff involved could be determined.

When these data were considered by grade of the first clinical reviewer at the hospital a clearer picture emerged and the percentage of inappropriate responses rose from 3.1% when consultants were the first reviewer to 23.5% when SHOs were the first reviewer.

Appropriateness of initial hospital response and overall care

Table 27 shows only those patients who were classified as having an inappropriate initial response (94/699 from Table 25). Only a handful of the cases (8/94) were graded as having good overall care. In addition 17/94 received less than satisfactory care in the view of the advisors.

Table 27 reflects the importance of the initial response in the view of the advisors; both in terms of clinical decision making, and overall care for the severely injured patient. If the initial in-hospital phase of trauma care is not good then the remainder of the patient journey is more likely to be sub-standard.

Key findings

Less than half (47.7%) of the patients in this study received good care.

Patients were more likely to receive good care in centres that reported a high volume of cases (>20) compared to a low volume of cases (<20) – 57% v 39%.

13.4% of cases had an inappropriate initial hospital response. It was much more likely to be an inappropriate response if the team leader/first reviewer was an SHO (23.5%) than a consultant (3.1%).

If the initial hospital response was inappropriate, it was more likely that the patient's overall care would be compromised.

CHAPTER 4 - Prehospital care

Introduction

The administration of high quality prehospital care is vital in any system of trauma care. Prioritisation and management of life threatening injuries, coupled with rapid transfer to definitive care in an appropriately equipped trauma unit are the mainstay of this phase of the trauma system. The emphasis on prehospital care versus rapid transfer varies between countries, with little evidence of one system having advantages over the other[1]. However, it must be emphasised that there is no dichotomy between prehospital care and rapid transfer as all care should be tailored to deal with the patient's injuries and any consequent physiological derangements. Patients undergoing rapid transfer must still receive appropriate prehospital care.

Trauma systems are primarily geared towards the management of small and manageable numbers of casualties, which do not overwhelm the local resources available. Special measures are required when the number of casualties exceeds the capacity of the local resources. In this event, a major incident will be declared, and a multi-agency predetermined major incident plan will be initiated. Such a plan is necessary to ensure a high standard of care is delivered to all patients presenting as part of a major incident. In this study there were 12 cases reported where it was indicated on the questionnaire that a "major incident" had occurred[2]. However, on more detailed examination of the casenotes, none of these cases arose in situations which fulfilled the requirements of the definition of a major incident and in no case was a major incident formally declared. Since none of the patients in this study were involved in a major incident, it would be expected that resources should have been sufficient to provide the usual standard of care.

As mentioned in the methods section, it had been hoped that some additional information regarding the prehospital management of patients could be obtained from a questionnaire completed by ambulance crews. However, it proved difficult to agree this with ambulance services, partly due to employment contract issues and partly due to the re-organisation of ambulance trusts.

Organisational aspects of care

Prehospital documentation

In a third of cases (245/749), the ambulance patient report form (PRF) was not available. Data in this chapter therefore refers to the 504 cases where a PRF was returned. This is an important healthcare record which provides treating clinicians with vital prehospital information regarding the incident and prehospital management. This form could also provide a structure to ensure that protocols of prehospital management are followed, and that data relevant to subsequent service audit are accurately recorded. Unfortunately, there was no uniformity between ambulance trusts; with wide variation in the content of PRFs. Appendix D demonstrates an example of an excellent PRF. It should be noted that the PRF is often a non-standard size which does not fit into the hospital casenotes and, therefore, it may become misplaced.

Response times

Response times from the time of the emergency call to arrival at the scene of accident varied. This information, analysed by time of day, is shown in Figure 6. The mean response time for day, evening and night was 12.5, 11.6 and 10.1 minutes respectively.

Overall there were better response times at night, although it is doubtful if this is of clinical relevance.

Response time and outcome

It is often said that rapid response times are essential and associated with better outcomes although it is difficult to find data to support this statement. Table 28 shows mortality rate at 72 hours post injury against response time.

In this study there was no clear evidence to support the association of response time with better outcome. Indeed the group with the fastest response time (0-5min) did not have a lower mortality than the rest of the population (Table 28).

Figure 6. Time from emergency call to scene of accident (daytime is defined as 08.00–17.59, evening from 18.00-23.59 and night time from 00.00-07.59)

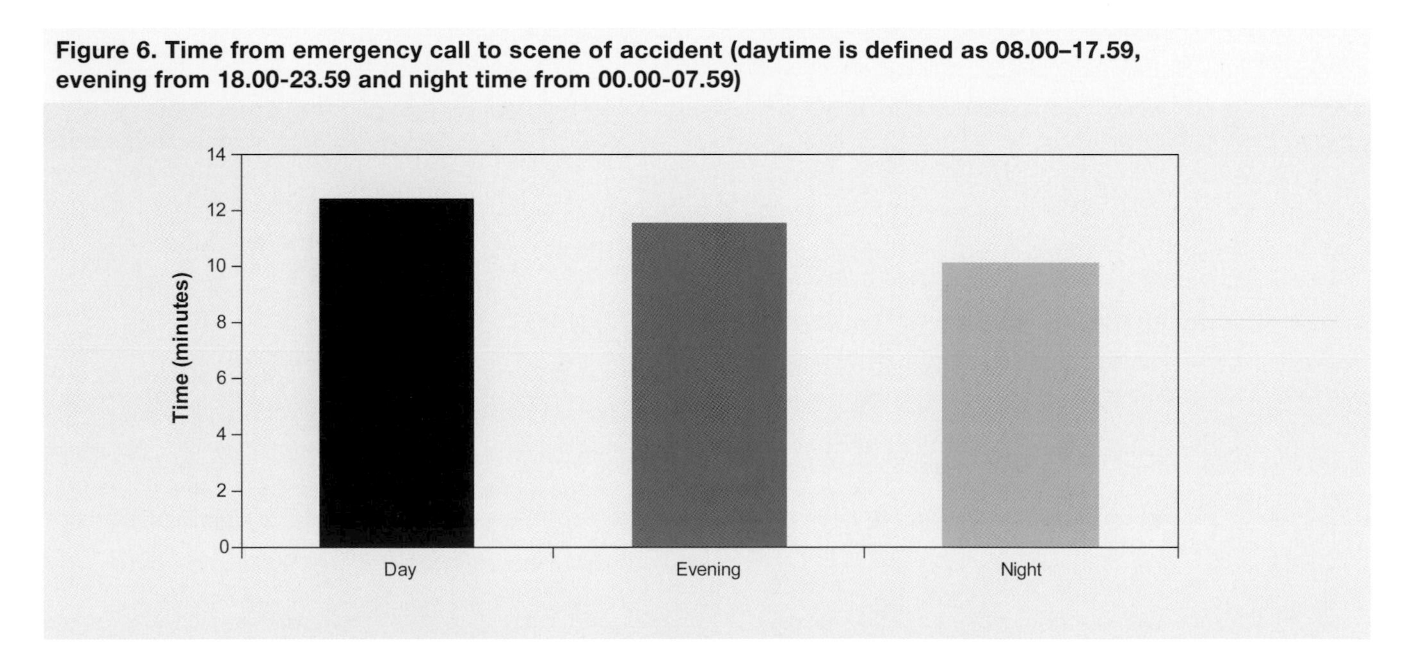

Table 28. Prehospital response times (minutes) and patient outcome at 72 hours

	Alive	Deceased	Total	% mortality
0-5	72	20	**92**	21.7
6-10	111	18	**129**	14.0
11-15	66	12	**78**	15.4
16-20	40	6	**46**	13.0
21-25	24	6	**30**	20.0
26-30	7	2	**9**	22.2
> 30	11	2	**13**	15.4

Mode of arrival

The mode of arrival is shown in Table 29.

Table 29. Mode of arrival

	Number of patients	%
Ambulance	652	83.3
Helicopter	92	11.7
Other emergency service	5	<1
Hospital transfer	9	1.1
Member of public	13	1.7
Self referral	8	1.0
Other	4	<1
Subtotal	**783**	
Not recorded	12	
Total	**795**	

Effect of time on mode of arrival

Figure 7 shows that helicopters were much less likely to be employed at night. Approximately 75% of helicopter transfers occurred during daytime hours.

Figure 7. The effect of time of day on the employment of helicopters (daytime was defined as 08.00–17.59 and night time from 18.00-07.59)

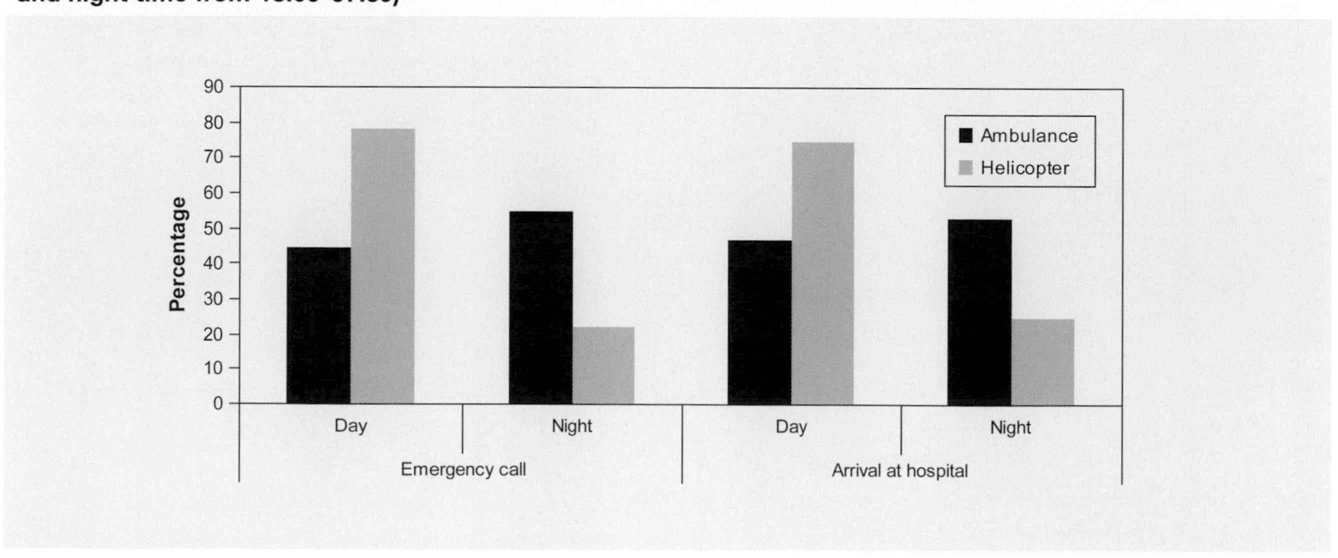

Figure 8. Length of time at scene of injury

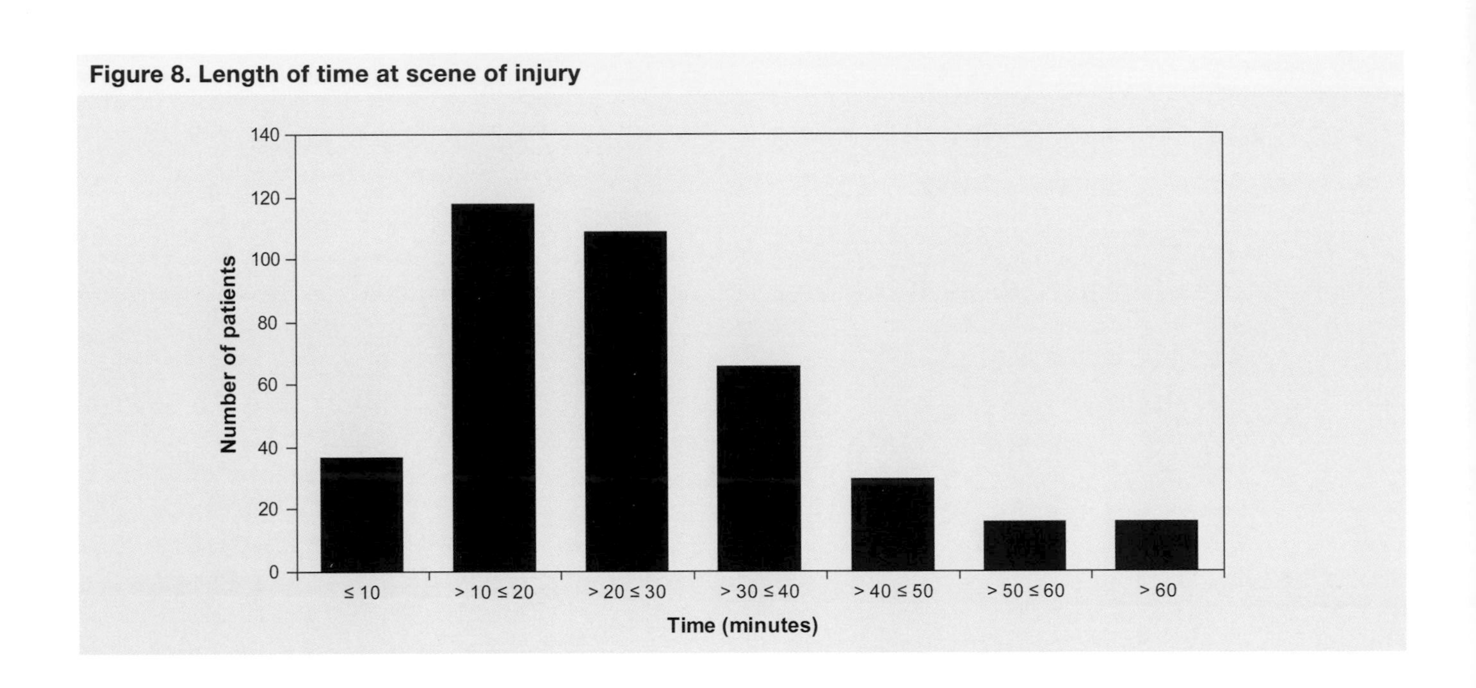

Time at scene

In those cases (386/504) where the timings could be determined, the vast majority (349), exceeded the recommended length of time on scene of 10 minutes[3] (Figure 8). In 71 cases delay was due to entrapment. Even if the entrapped were excluded, 278 cases exceeded 10 minutes at the scene. In a further 105 cases either intubation and/or cannulation were undertaken at the scene, and these manoeuvres may have contributed to the extended time at the scene. The 10 minute on scene recommendation refers to paramedic care and in the presence of a prehospital physician system (where more interventions are likely, e.g. tracheal intubation) a longer time is probably justifiable.

Transport system and prehospital timings

The role of helicopters in the management of trauma patients remains controversial[4]. Some trauma victims may benefit but others may not. Previous studies in the USA have suggested that total times from alert to arrival at hospital are significantly longer in all types of location by helicopter as opposed to road ambulance[5].

There was a greater time to reach hospital from the time of the emergency call, and an increased time spent at the scene of the incident, for those patients transported by helicopter (Figure 9).

The longer time spent at the scene for patients transported by helicopter could, in part, be attributed to the greater likelihood of there being a doctor on the scene, and of the patient being intubated before transfer. We were unable to identify which cases were attended by doctors or paramedics.

Figure 9. Average response times and time at scene: ambulance vs. helicopter

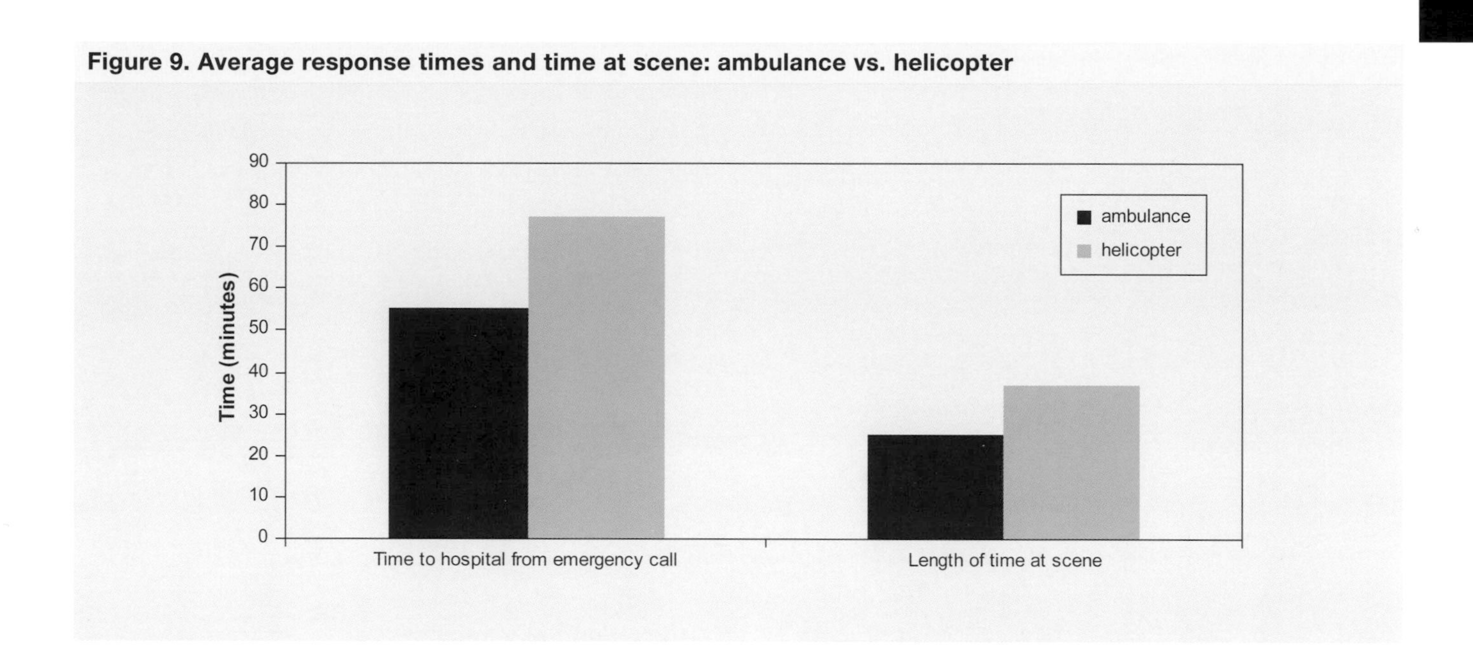

Transport system and prehospital airway management

From the cases where it could be determined, 23/56 (41.1%) patients transported by helicopter were intubated at the scene versus 32/440 (7.3%) of those patients transported by ambulance. Additionally it was found that a greater percentage of patients transported by ambulance arrived at hospital with a noisy or blocked airway compared with those transported by helicopter (52/380; 13.7% v 3/54; 5.6%). Patients treated and transferred by a helicopter system had a greater chance of definitive airway control than those treated and transferred by a road ambulance system.

Transport system and severity of injuries

The severity of injuries in both groups was comparable (Table 30).

Table 30. Transport system by injury severity score

	Road ambulance		Helicopter	
ISS	Number of patients	%	Number of patients	%
16 - 24	240	54.5	31	52.5
25 - 35	156	35.5	20	33.9
36 - 75	44	10.0	8	13.6
Total	**440**		**59**	

Transport system and secondary transfer rate

The likelihood of requiring a secondary transfer was lower if the patient's mode of arrival was by helicopter than for those patients who arrived by road ambulance. Only 7/59 (11.9%) patients required a secondary transfer in the helicopter group compared with 112/440 (25.5%) transported initially by road ambulance.

Transport system and appropriateness of initial hospital

It was judged that all of the patients transported by helicopter were taken to an appropriate hospital. However, it was deemed that 31/440 (7%) patients transported by road ambulance were taken to an inappropriate first hospital.

Transport systems – summary

Overall, the picture regarding mode of transport is complex. There is a potential danger in making assumptions regarding the appropriateness of the mode of transport in any individual case if conclusions are drawn from aggregated data derived from a heterogeneous population. Helicopters should not only be considered as a mode of transport, but also as a system of care with the potential to deliver rapidly to the scene of the incident a doctor with sufficient expertise to manage these challenging patients. However, given the significant expense involved in operating helicopters, it is important that a careful and detailed audit of the value of helicopter transport is undertaken.

In summary, helicopter transport was used for 11.7% of the severely injured patients in this study, with most episodes taking place in daylight hours. Treatment and transport by a helicopter-based team compared to a ground ambulance-based team was associated with a longer on scene time (36.9 minutes v 25.3 minutes) and a longer total prehospital time (77.4mins v 55.2mins). However, the patient was more likely to be intubated (41.1% v 7.3%), less likely to arrive at hospital with a completely or partially blocked airway, more likely to be triaged to an appropriate hospital (100% v 93%) and less likely to require a secondary transfer (11.9% v 25.5%).

Clinical aspects of care

Primary and secondary survey

In the majority of patients, a primary survey was conducted at the site of the incident, en route or at some unspecified stage prior to arrival at hospital.

Table 31. Primary and secondary survey performed

	Primary		Secondary	
		%		%
Yes at scene	248	52.4	169	60.6
Yes en route	5	1.1	30	10.8
Yes unknown	220	46.5	80	28.7
Subtotal	**473**		**279**	
Not recorded	31		225	
Total	**504**		**504**	

However, in 31/504 (6.2%) cases, there was no record of a primary survey having been completed (Table 31).

In 199/504 cases a secondary survey was known to have been performed in the prehospital phase. In nearly half of cases the secondary survey was not recorded.

It is not clear why so many patients had a secondary survey performed, as the priority in the prehospital phase should be a good primary survey and attention to any immediate problems with the airway, cervical spine, breathing and circulation as the prime focus. Repeated evaluation of these aspects of care is required en route to hospital and while a secondary survey may provide valuable information regarding the patient's overall condition, it must not distract from this.

Airway and ventilation

Airway status at scene

In 85/504 cases it was recorded that the airway was either partially (noisy) or completely obstructed (blocked) (Table 32).

Table 32. Airway status

	Number of patients	%
Clear	343	80.1
Noisy	46	10.7
Blocked	39	9.1
Subtotal	**428**	
Not recorded	76	
Total	**504**	

Prehospital intubation

Twenty two of the patients with airway obstruction were intubated at the scene. Attempted intubation failed in six patients at the scene but all were successfully intubated in the emergency department. A further 34 patients, for whom the airway status was clear or not recorded, were intubated at the scene (56 in total). However, three more failed attempts were documented in this group.

Monitoring and oxygen therapy

The respiratory rate is an important indicator of respiratory function and of shock. Respiratory rate was not recorded in 65/504 (13%) patients (Figure 10).

Oxygen therapy was administered to 372/504 (73.8%) patients, but was not documented as being administered in the remaining 132 cases. The use of assisted ventilation was poorly documented.

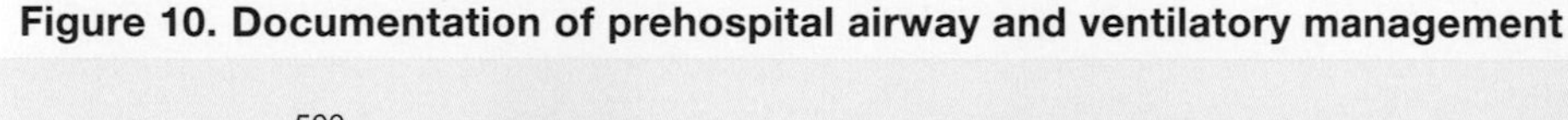

Figure 10. Documentation of prehospital airway and ventilatory management

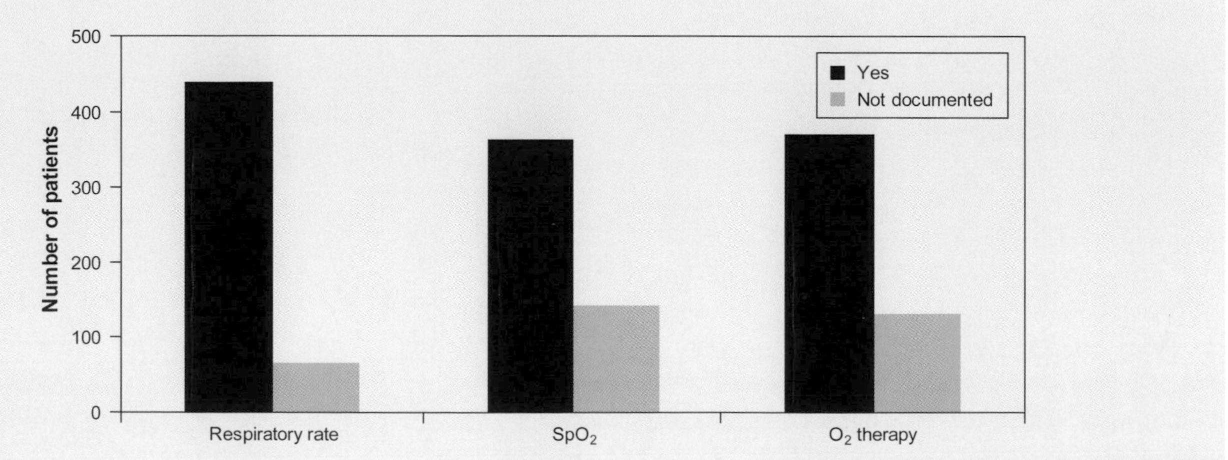

Adequacy of prehospital airway and ventilation

Tables 33 and 34 show the advisors' opinion on prehospital airway and ventilation management.

Table 33. Adequate airway secured

	Number of patients	%
Yes	396	90.4
No	42	9.6
Subtotal	**438**	
Insufficient data	66	
Total	**504**	

Table 34. Adequate ventilation secured

	Number of patients	%
Yes	401	92.0
No	35	8.0
Subtotal	**436**	
Insufficient data	68	
Total	**504**	

The advisors were of the opinion that airway management in the prehospital phase was inadequate in 42 out of the 438 cases that could be assessed. In a number of these cases (12/42), it was felt that prehospital intubation should have been attempted. In 35/436 (8%) cases, advisors felt that ventilation was inadequate. NCEPOD did not request any data on the use of capnography in the prehospital phase.

The management of the airway and breathing in the prehospital setting is currently the responsibility of paramedics because very few areas in the UK have a system of care that ensures a doctor is part of the response team. Whilst it is not current practice for paramedics to routinely perform tracheal intubation on trauma patients, they may undertake this task when the airway is compromised and basic airway manoeuvres have failed. Paramedics in Britain do not use anaesthetic drugs or muscle relaxants to achieve intubation and, therefore, can only attempt this in the most obtunded patients.

The literature points to a high mortality in the prehospital phase when trauma patients are intubated without the need for anaesthesia[6, 7]. This probably reflects the severity of their injuries, in that they can tolerate laryngoscopy and intubation without anaesthesia, rather than the effect of the procedure itself.

The literature is confusing with regards to the effects of prehospital intubation of trauma patients. Some studies have shown increased mortality whilst others have shown benefit[8-11]. It is difficult to separate the effects of underlying injuries, anaesthesia, skill and experience of the intubator from the possible benefits or side effects of the procedure.

A recent expert panel concluded that suboptimal anaesthetic technique as well as subsequent hyperventilation may account for some of the mortality reported with prehospital airway management in systems where anaesthesia is available[12].

Invasive airway management at the scene is successfully performed in systems that supply physician staffed ambulances, and is considered a vital part of their advanced trauma life support[10, 13, 14].

As can be seen, there is little high quality evidence to support either opinion. Most of the studies favouring prehospital endotracheal intubation of severely traumatised patients were conducted in out-of-hospital systems that rely on highly skilled personnel such as anaesthetists, emergency physicians, or specially trained nurses, mostly in continental Europe or Australia. In contrast, studies that do not support this approach rely on data from paramedic or emergency technician staffed services, mostly in the USA or the UK. The conclusion must be that if prehospital intubation is to be part of prehospital trauma management then it needs to be in the context of a physician-based prehospital care system.

Figure 11. Documentation of prehospital cardiovascular measurements

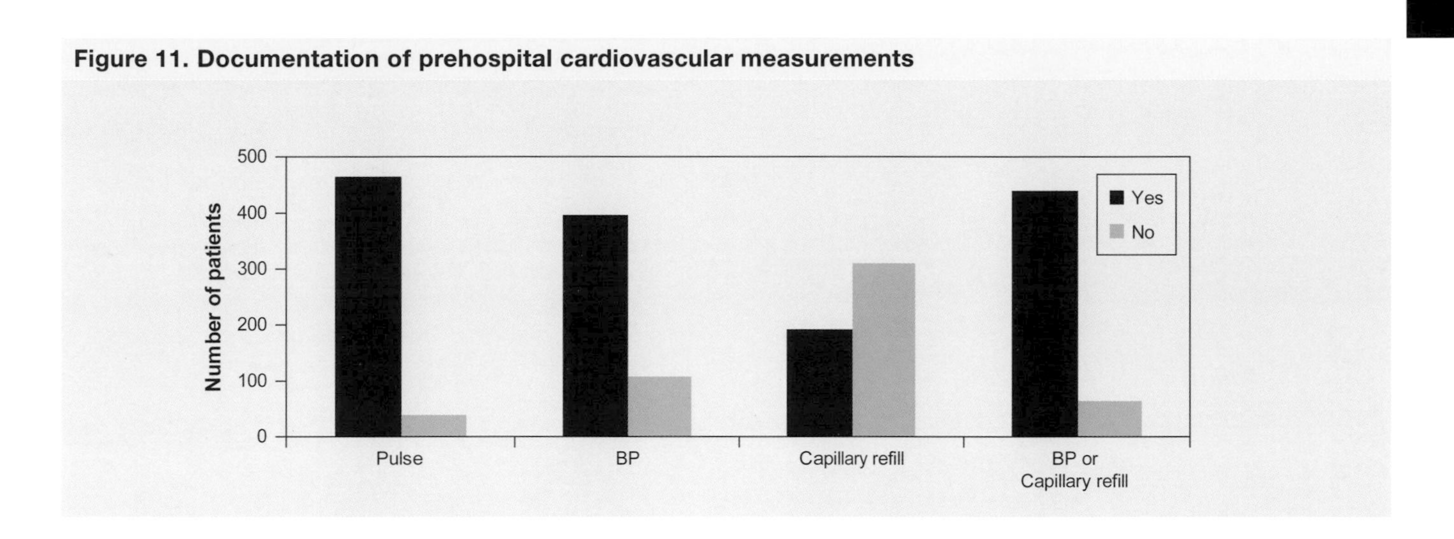

Cardiovascular management

There are two sets of recommendations and guidelines in relation to this that are closely interlinked: The National Institute for Health and Clinical Excellence (NICE) and Joint Royal Colleges Ambulance Liaison Committee (JRCALC). Prehospital staff are more likely to be familiar with JRCALC guidelines, and hospital staff more familiar with NICE recommendations, which are in fact published as a technology appraisal[16], not as clinical guidelines.

The recommendations arising from the NICE technology appraisal, and included within the JRCALC guidelines[15], are as follows:

> "It is recommended that in the prehospital management of adults and older children, IV fluid should not be administered if a radial pulse can be felt (or, for penetrating torso injuries, if a central pulse can be felt).
>
> In the absence of a radial pulse (or a central pulse for penetrating torso injuries) in adults and older children, it is recommended that IV fluid should be administered in boluses of no more than 250 ml. The patient should then be reassessed, and the process repeated until a radial pulse (or central pulse for penetrating torso injuries) is palpable.
>
> The administration of IV fluid should not delay transportation to hospital, but when given in accordance with the recommendation above, consideration should be given to administration en route to hospital.
>
> It is recommended that when IV fluid is indicated in the prehospital setting, crystalloid solutions should be the routine choice.
>
> There is inadequate evidence on which the Institute can base recommendations on when prehospital use of IV fluid in young children and infants following trauma is appropriate, or on the volumes of fluid to use. However, there is a broad consensus that transfer to hospital should not be delayed by attempts to administer IV fluid.
>
> It is recommended that only healthcare professionals who have been appropriately trained in advanced life-support techniques and prehospital care should administer IV fluid therapy to trauma patients in the prehospital setting.
>
> Training programmes for healthcare professionals should incorporate the above recommendations."

In 40/504 (7.9%) cases the pulse was not recorded. Blood pressure was recorded in 398/504 (78.9%) cases. 21/504 (4.2%) patients did not have any measurements of their cardiovascular status recorded prior to arrival at hospital.

Measurement of blood pressure at the site of incident or en route, is not recommended particularly in children, as it may lead to unnecessary delay.

Fluid therapy was recorded as being administered either at the scene or en route in 188/504 cases.

Table 35. Appropriate haemorrhage control (advisors' opinion)

	Number of patients	%
Yes	356	96.7
No	12	3.3
Subtotal	**368**	
Insufficient data	136	
Total	**504**	

Table 36. Appropriate fluid therapy (advisors' opinion)

	Number of patients	%
Yes	279	87.2
No	41	12.8
Subtotal	**320**	
Insufficient data	184	
Total	**504**	

The advisors assessed that in 12 cases, insufficient steps had been taken to control haemorrhage (Table 35), and in 41 cases fluids were not administered appropriately (Table 36). In most cases this was because inadequate volumes, or in some cases no fluid, was administered, despite clinical features of shock. However, there were no cases in which the advisors believed that children under the age of 16 years had received inappropriate fluid resuscitation prehospital.

Head injury

In 25 cases the Glasgow Coma Score (GCS) or AVPU (Alert, Verbal, Pain, Unresponsive) score was not recorded

Figure 12. Prehospital Glasgow Coma Score (GCS)

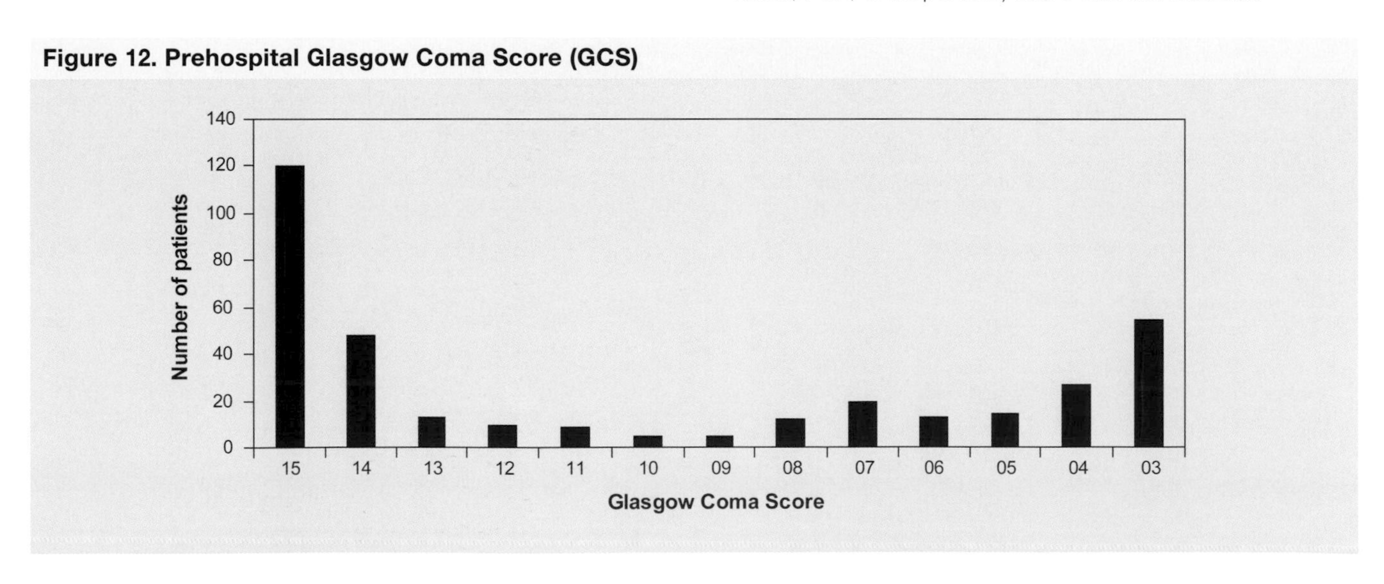

Figure 13. Prehospital Glasgow Coma Score and intubation

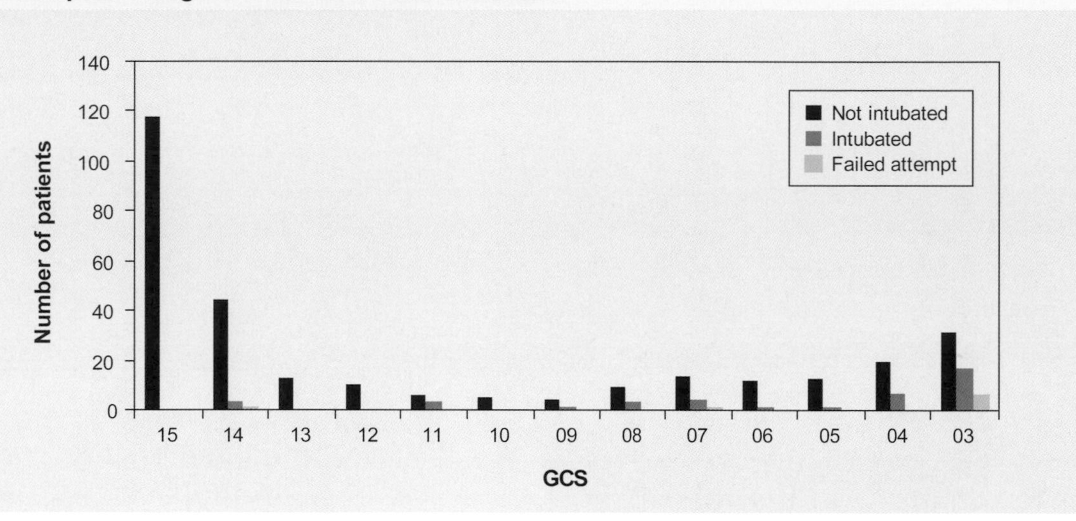

(Table 37). This could be taken to mean that the score was normal. However, it is important that the GCS or AVPU is recorded, so that any deterioration later in the patient journey can be clearly and unequivocally identified.

Where the airway was at risk because of a GCS less than 9, intubation was performed in only 46/170 patients. Documentation of other forms of assisted ventilation was noted to be poor. Advisors considered that the airway/ventilatory management could have been better in a substantial number of patients, a number of whom had a lowered GCS (Figure 13 and Table 38). Many patients who may have benefited from intubation did not have this procedure performed because the appropriate skills were not available.

Analgesia

The administration of analgesia prehospital was documented in 110/504 cases. The advisors considered that the analgesia was inappropriate for 7/110 of these cases. In one such case it was felt that an overdose had been administered. In another case the administration of analgesia

Table 37. Prehospital AVPU score

Alert	68
Verbal	21
Pain	17
Unresponsive	21
Subtotal	**127**
GCS or AVPU not recorded	25
Total	**152**

Table 38. Prehospital AVPU score and intubation

	Not intubated	Intubated	Failed attempt
Alert	0	0	0
Verbal	0	0	0
Pain	11	5	1
Unresponsive	13	8	0
Total	**26**	**13**	**1**

caused respiratory depression which was not adequately managed by suitable respiratory support. In three cases with significant thoracic injuries Entonox was the analgesic used and this was considered by the advisors to be inappropriate because of the risk of tension pneumothorax.

One must question why the provision of analgesia in a group of severely injured patients was so low (110/504 – 21.8%)? Patients with severe injuries are likely to experience pain and the provision of analgesia to reduce this is a basic humanitarian aim. It is rare that contraindications exist to the provision of pain relief.

Key findings

In a third of cases (245/749), the ambulance patient report form was not available.

652/783 patients (83.3%) were transported to hospital by road ambulance and 92/783 patients (11.7%) by helicopter.

23/56 (41.1%) patients treated by a helicopter-based system were intubated on scene compared to 32/440 (7.3%) patients treated by a road ambulance system.

None of the patients treated by a helicopter based system were taken to an inappropriate hospital compared to 31/440 (7%) patients treated by a road ambulance system who were initially taken to an inappropriate hospital.

Blood pressure was recorded in 398/504 (80%) cases despite recommendations that this should not be measured in the prehospital phase.

Only 46/170 (27.1%) patients who suffered a severe head injury (GCS less than 9) were intubated prehospital.

Only 110/504 (21.8%) patients were given analgesia in the prehospital phase.

Recommendations

All agencies involved in trauma management, including emergency medical services, should be integrated into the clinical governance programmes of a regional trauma service. *(All healthcare providers)*

Ambulance trusts should work together to standardise the content and layout of the Patient Report Form (PRF), and ensure that it is fit for purpose and facilitates comparative audit. Clinicians must ensure that a PRF is received for every patient and secured in the medical record. *(Emergency medicine physicians and ambulance crews)*

It is important that where guidelines exist, they are widely disseminated to appropriate groups, and there is a robust system in place to monitor compliance with those guidelines. *(Ambulance and hospital trusts)*

It is vital that all patients who have sustained serious trauma should have a primary survey conducted at the earliest opportunity, and that critical resuscitation involving airway, breathing and circulation (with cervical spine control) should be undertaken and reviewed throughout the prehospital phase of care. This must be documented. *(Emergency medicine physicians)*

Airway management in trauma patients is often challenging. The prehospital response for these patients should include someone with the skill to secure the airway, (including the use of rapid sequence intubation), and maintain adequate ventilation. *(Ambulance and hospital trusts)*

Severely injured patients are likely to be in pain and the provision of adequate analgesia is required. If analgesia is not given there should be a clear record in the Patient Report Form of the reasons for this. *(Ambulance trusts)*

References

1. Nathens AB, Brunet FP, Maier RV. *Development of trauma systems and effect on outcomes after injury.* Lancet 2004; 363(9423):1794-801

2. The form sent to lead A&E Clinicians contained the following definition of a major incident protocol: "Pre-planned and exercised procedures which are activated once a major incident has been declared. A major incident is any emergency that requires the implementation of special arrangements by one or more emergency services, the NHS or the local authority".

3. The Royal College of Surgeons of England and the British Orthopaedic Society. *Better Care for the Severely Injured.* 2000

4. Thomas SH, Biddinger PD, *Helicopter trauma transport: an overview of recent outcomes and triage literature.* Current Opinion in Anaesthesiology 2003; 16(2):153-8

5. Carr BG, Caplan JM, Pryor JP, Branas CC. *A meta-analysis of prehospital care times for trauma.* Prehospital Emergency Care 2006; 10(2):198-206

6. Lockey D, Davies G, Coats T. *Survival of trauma patients who have prehospital tracheal intubation without anaesthesia or muscle relaxants: observational study.* BMJ 2001; 323:141

7. Christensen EF, Hoyer CC. *Prehospital tracheal intubation in severely injured patients: a Danish observational study.* BMJ 2003; 327:533-4

8. Winchell RJ, Hoyt DB: *Endotracheal intubation in the field improves survival in patients with severe head injury.* Trauma Research and Education Foundation of San Diego. Arch Surg 1997; 132:592-7

9. Garner A, Rashford S, Lee A, Bartolacci R. *Addition of physicians to paramedic helicopter services decreases blunt trauma mortality.* Aust N Z J Surg 1999; 69:697-701

10. Adnet F, Jouriles NJ, Le Toumelin P, Hennequin B, Taillandier C, Rayeh F, Couvreur J, Nougiere B, Nadiras P, Ladka A, Fleury M: *Survey of out-of-hospital emergency intubations in the French prehospital medical system: a multicenter study.* Ann Emerg Med 1998; 32:454-60

11. Bochicchio GV, Ilahi O, Joshi M, Bochicchio K, Scalea TM. *Endotracheal intubation in the field does not improve outcome in trauma patients who present without an acutely lethal traumatic brain injury.* J Trauma 2003; 54:307-11

12. Davis DP, Fakhry SM, Wang HE, Bulger EM, Domeier RM, Trask AL, Bochiocchio GV, Hauda WE, Robinsion L. *Paramedic rapid sequence intubation for severe traumatic brain injury: perspectives from an expert panel.* Prehosp Emerg Care 2007; 11:1-8

13. Gerich TG, Schmidt U, Hubrich V, Lobenhoffer HP, Tscherne H: *Prehospital airway management in the acutely injured patient: the role of surgical cricothyrotomy revisited.* J Trauma 1998; 45:312-4

14. Schmidt U, Frame SB, Nerlich ML, Rowe DW, Enderson BL, Maull KI, Tscherne H: *On-scene helicopter transport of patients with multiple injuries: comparison of a German and an American system.* J Trauma 1992; 33:548-53

15. UK Ambulance Service Clinical Practice Guidelines 2006. Joint Royal Colleges Ambulance Liaison Committee (JRCALC)

16. NICE Technology Appraisal. Prehospital initiation of fluid replacement therapy in trauma. 2004

CHAPTER 5 - Hospital reception

Introduction

Deaths after major trauma can be grouped into immediate, early, and late deaths.

Immediate deaths are caused by a fatal disruption of the great vessels, heart, lungs or a major disruption of body cavities. Immediate death occurs at the scene of injury. This group of deaths is least likely to be influenced by measures taken post injury. Injury prevention strategies and public health measures must remain the major strategy for reducing this major source of mortality.

Early deaths occur in the hours just after the injury. These patients frequently arrive at a hospital prior to death which usually occurs because of cardiovascular and/or pulmonary collapse. Early trauma deaths result from failed oxygenation of the vital organs, massive central nervous system injury, or both. The mechanisms of failed tissue oxygenation include inadequate ventilation, impaired oxygenation, circulatory collapse, and insufficient end-organ perfusion. Injuries that cause early trauma mortality occur in predictable patterns based on the mechanism of injury; the patient's age, gender, and body habitus; or environmental conditions. Rapid resuscitation coupled with rapid definitive management of injuries and complications has the potential to reduce these deaths.

Late deaths peak from days to weeks after the injury and are due primarily to sepsis and multiple organ failure.

Organised systems for trauma care are often thought to be focused on the salvage of a patient from early trauma mortality, while critical care is designed to manage complications and avert late trauma mortality. However, it must be noted that a good trauma process (early definitive care and optimal resuscitation) will not only reduce early mortality but also reduce the number of late deaths by minimising the number of patients who go on to develop multiple organ failure and require critical care. Importantly from the perspective of survivors, a good trauma process may also reduce morbidity.

The recognition of these patterns led to the development of the advanced trauma life support (ATLS) approach by the American College of Surgeons. ATLS is the basis of trauma care and it is built around a standardised protocol for patient evaluation. This protocol ensures that the most immediate life-threatening conditions are actively identified and addressed in the order of their risk potential.

The objectives of the initial evaluation of the trauma patient are:

1. to identify life-threatening injuries and to initiate adequate supportive therapy;
2. to efficiently and rapidly organise either definitive therapy or transfer to a facility that provides definitive therapy.

This chapter describes the initial reception of the severely injured patient and organisation of the trauma response.

Results

Pre-alerts

From the introduction above it can be appreciated that one of the key steps in maximising outcome for the severely injured patient is to ensure a rapid and appropriate emergency department response. One mechanism for ensuring that this occurs is communication from the prehospital clinicians to the receiving emergency department, passing on details of the extent of the injuries and the response required in hospital. This communication is referred to as a pre-alert.

Figure 14. Documentation of a pre-alert (daytime was defined as 08.00–17.59, evening from 18.00-23.59 and night time from 00.00-07.59)

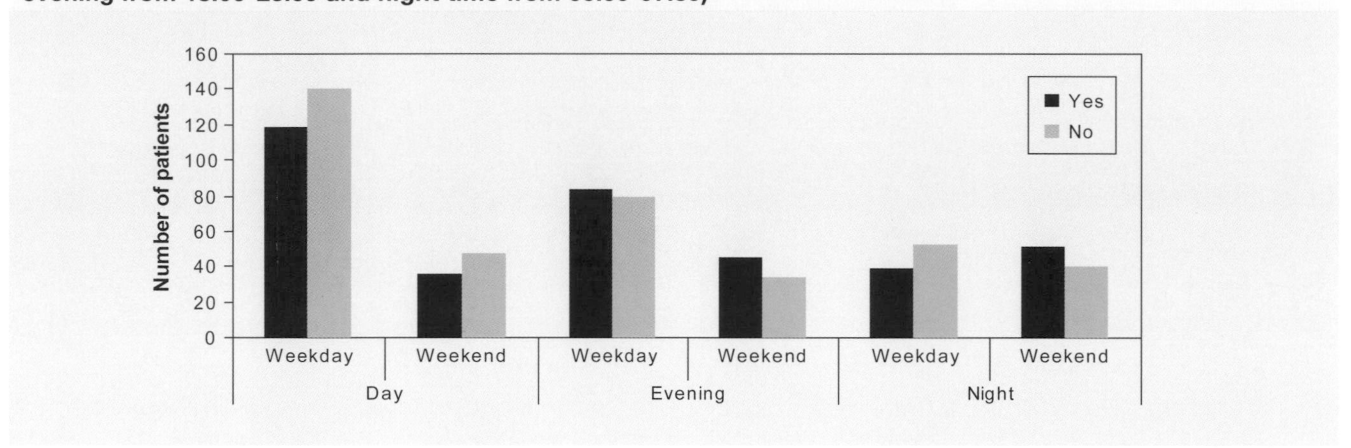

Documentation of ambulance pre-alert

As can be seen from Figure 14 the use of pre-alerts was quite low with only 50.1% (375/749) of the patients arriving at hospital with a pre-alert. It does not appear that the time of day, nor day of week, affected the use of pre-alerts to any great extent.

It has previously been recommended that all hospitals that receive patients following major injury should establish a system of advance notification with the ambulance service[1]. This arrangement should allow the ambulance paramedic at the scene to notify the emergency department directly of the details of the injured patient(s). The aim of pre-alerts is to anticipate and be prepared for problems so that resuscitation, investigation and definitive management can proceed with minimum delay.

Worthy of note was the fact that the use of pre-alerts was so infrequent in this dataset; particularly in view of the fact that only patients with a verified injury severity score (ISS) score of 16 or greater were included in this study. It is likely that the low use of pre-alerts may slow down an appropriate initial response to these severely injured patients and delay definitive care, especially as we have seen that senior trauma team leaders were often not immediately available.

Trauma team response

It is essential for each hospital that admits major trauma cases to have a trauma response team[1]. The initial management of the trauma patient can be extremely challenging and requires a co-ordinated team approach to deliver timely and correct treatment to these patients. Each hospital and the ambulance service should also agree criteria for activation of the trauma team. Ideally this should occur prior to the patient's arrival in the resuscitation room.

Trauma team response – organisational aspects

Of the 183 sites that submitted an organisational questionnaire 143 (78.1%) had a formal trauma team. All but nine of these had a written protocol for activation of the trauma team.

Table 39. Trauma respondents by grade of specialty

	Consultant		Emergency Medicine SpR or above		Anaesthetic SpR or above		Surgical SpR or above	
		%		%		%		%
Resident	6	3.3	109	59.6	111	60.7	86	47.0
Non-resident	59	32.2	36	19.7	13	7.1	34	18.6
Not present	118	64.5	38	20.8	59	32.2	63	34.4
Total	**183**		**183**		**183**		**183**	

It has previously been shown that only half of the emergency departments attending more than 30 000 patients per year operated a trauma team system[2]. A more recent study has shown some improvement in availability of trauma teams with 61% of departments surveyed operating such a system[3]. The availability of trauma teams has continued to increase and that the figure now approaches 80%. However, one in five departments in this study, despite accepting severely injured patients, did not have a formal trauma team. This is presumably an issue of organisation as these departments should have the necessary personnel but for some reason had not arranged their activity into a structured trauma response.

As part of the organisational questionnaire NCEPOD requested information about who would respond to a request for a trauma response in the early hours of a Sunday morning (0200). Table 39 shows the response analysed by grade and availability.

One hundred and eighteen of the 183 (65%) hospitals from which an organisational questionnaire was received responded that a consultant would not be present during the trauma call. There were also a number of hospitals where it was stated that they would not have the presence of a SpR or above from the emergency department (38/183; 20.8%), anaesthesia (59/183; 32.2%) or surgery (63/183; 34.4%).

There are clear recommendations regarding the composition of a trauma team: consultant leadership plus the presence of SpRs or above from the emergency department, anaesthesia and surgery are probably the key elements[1]. Table 39 shows that the current provision of staff falls well short of these recommendations.

In the hospitals where SpRs or above were either not present or non-resident, the initial care was presumably provided by more junior members of staff. This is a concern, as initial management may have a substantial impact on eventual outcome.

Immediate airway control is vital. Only 111/183 (60.7%) hospitals had an anaesthetic SpR or above immediately available. Trauma airways are likely to be difficult and a SpR or above should be present immediately.

Trauma team response - individual cases

Documentation of trauma team response

Figure 15 shows the trauma response analysed by time of day and weekday/weekend. Overall there was documentation of a trauma team response in 59.7% (460/770) of cases. In 25 cases there was insufficient data

Figure 15. Documentation of trauma response (daytime was defined as 08.00–17.59, evening from 18.00-23.59 and night time from 00.00-07.59)

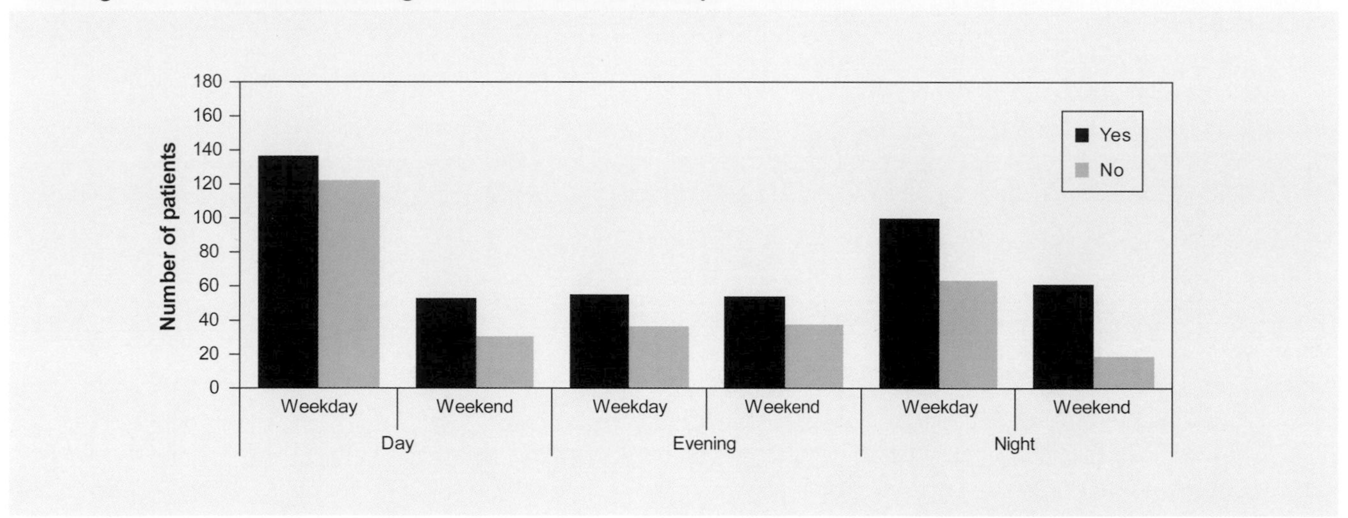

to determine if there was a trauma response. There was some variation in the activation of the trauma team by time of day and day of week. The trauma team was less likely to be present on a weekday during the day (137/259; 52.9%) than at nights (100/163; 61.3%) and weekends (168/256; 65.6%).

Possible explanations for the variation in trauma team response are:

1. Less need for a trauma team during the normal working day as there was an appropriate consultant response, and supporting team, immediately available within the receiving emergency department.

2. The trauma team had other responsibilities during the working day and so was less likely to be available to attend the emergency department for daytime trauma calls.

Influence of the severity of injury on the use of trauma teams

Table 40 describes the influence of the severity of injury and the initiation of a trauma team response. There was a trend towards greater involvement of trauma teams for patients with more severe injuries.

Table 40. Trauma call documented by ISS

	Trauma call documented		
ISS	**Yes**	**No**	**Total**
16 - 24	231	218	**449**
25 - 35	185	94	**279**
36 - 75	55	12	**67**
Total	**471**	**324**	**795**

While this may appear reassuring it must be remembered that this score was calculated retrospectively and cannot drive real time management decisions. Also many patients with an ISS in the range 16-24 can pose great challenges and do require the input of a well-organised trauma service.

Trauma team response to pre-alerts

The use of pre-alerts and activation of the trauma team are key initial components of an organised trauma system. Figure 16 shows the relationship between these two elements (data from A&E clinician questionnaire). It can be seen that even in the presence of a pre-alert there was no trauma team response in 99/383 (25.8%) cases.

The reasons for the lack of trauma team response to a pre-alert were not clear but in a substantial number of cases (99/383), where the prehospital clinicians had sufficient concerns to issue a pre-alert, no trauma team was activated.

Figure 16. Trauma team activation in response to pre-alert

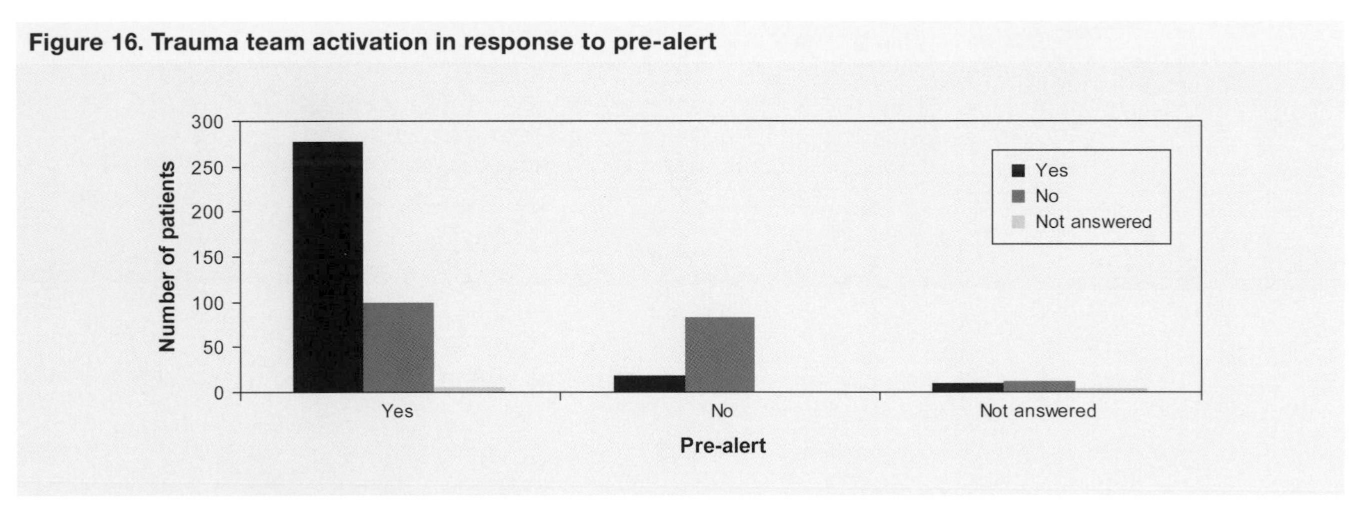

Figure 17. Grade of first reviewer/team leader in response to trauma call

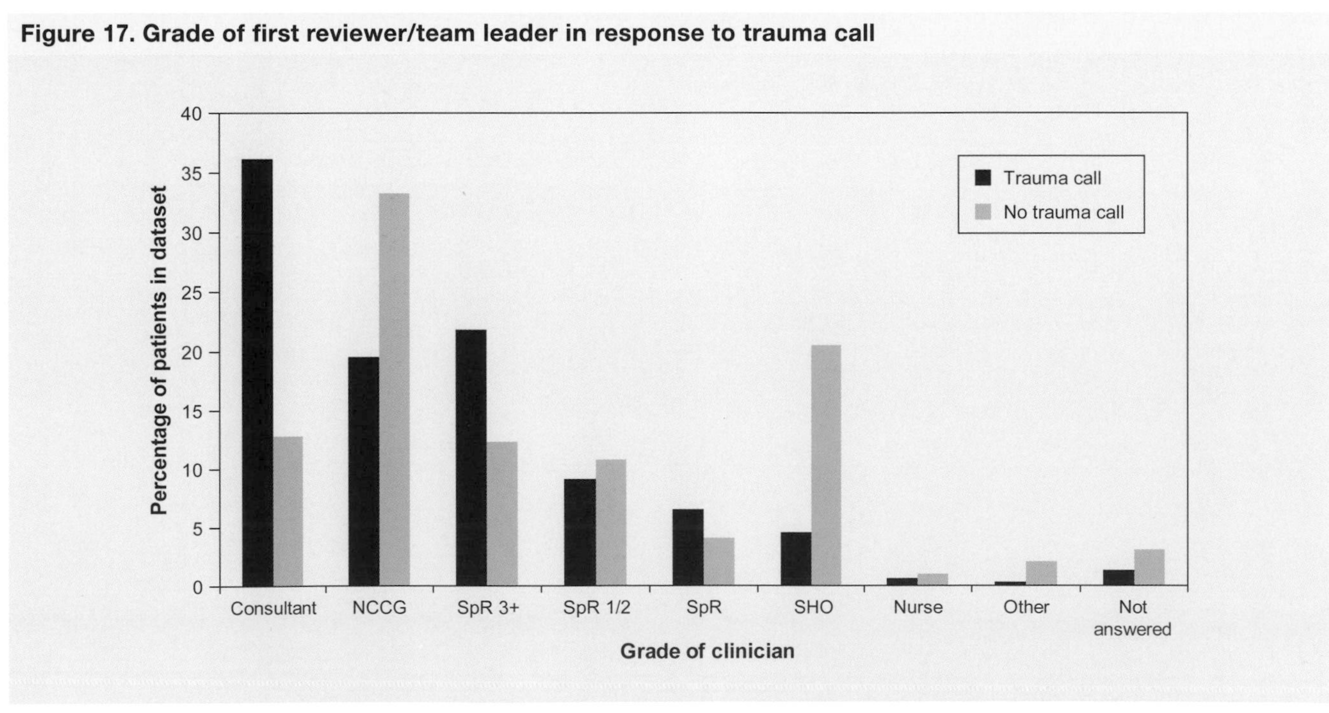

Trauma team leadership

The recommendations for an organised trauma response states that the trauma team leader must be a consultant from a relevant specialty[1], recognising that the management of the severely injured patient is potentially very challenging and requires considerable skill and experience.

Figure 17 shows the grade of first reviewer/team leader analysed by whether or not a trauma call had been made. A consultant was the team leader/first reviewer in 136 out of 502 cases (27%). An SHO was the team leader/first reviewer in 54 out of 502 cases (10.8%). In 11 cases the grade of reviewer was not answered.

Two other main findings emerge from these data.

1. If a trauma call had been made it was much more likely that a consultant was the first reviewer/team leader. Consultants were team leaders in 36.2% (111/307) of cases where a trauma call was made compared to only 12.8% (25/195) of cases where no trauma call was made.

2. If a trauma call had not been made it was much more likely that an SHO was the first reviewer/team leader. SHOs were team leaders in 20.5% (40/195) of cases where no trauma call was made compared to only 4.6% (14/307) of cases where a trauma call was made.

It was also noted from the A&E clinician questionnaire that 176/513 (34.3%) patients were not seen by a consultant from any specialty while in the emergency department. For a further 53/513 (10%) patients, the clinician completing this questionnaire was unable to determine what time the patient was first seen by a consultant in the emergency department.

The above data highlights the data shown earlier regarding the variability of trauma team response by time and day (Figure 15). If the trauma team was called less frequently during the day because the emergency department was appropriately staffed by consultants, then the proportion of consultants seeing patients where a trauma team was not called would be much higher and the involvement of SHOs lower. This was not the case. The above data supports the view that the response rate of the trauma team during normal working hours was lower than out of hours as the team had competing commitments during the normal working day and was not always available to attend trauma calls.

Junior medical staff were still the first reviewer/team leader in a substantial number of cases. Indeed, an SHO was the first reviewer/team leader in 54/502 (10.8%) cases. However, it appears that progress has been made in this aspect since 1992 when an SHO was in charge of initial hospital resuscitation in 826 out of 1445 patients with an ISS of 16 or greater (57.2%)[4]. While this progress is encouraging, it is important to recognise the challenge that the severely injured patient poses and that it is inappropriate for very junior medical staff to lead their care.

Time to consultant review

Given the current staffing of emergency departments it is clear that not all patients can be seen and assessed immediately by a consultant. In the absence of immediate consultant involvement timely review is required. Table 41 shows time to consultant involvement. Fifty percent of patients (210/419) were either seen immediately or within 30 minutes. However, 42% (176/419) were not seen by a consultant (of any specialty) in the emergency department and in a further 94 cases the time interval was not known or not answered.

Table 41. Consultant involvement

	Number of patients	%
On arrival	169	40.3
> 0 ≤ 30 minutes	41	9.8
> 30 minutes	33	7.9
Not seen by consultant	176	42.0
Subtotal	**419**	
Time unknown	59	
Not answered	35	
Total	**513**	

These data are taken directly from the A&E clinician questionnaire (self reported) and as such should not suffer from the difficulty of obtaining information from the casenotes (where poor documentation often hinders assessment of staff involvement).

The time to consultant involvement was analysed by ISS, to see if consultants were more likely to be involved early in more severely injured patients. There was no influence of ISS on time to consultant involvement.

Impact of time of day on grade of reviewer

Another way to analyse the data on grade of the first reviewer/team leader was to consider the impact of time of day of presentation to the emergency department. These data are summarised in Table 42.

From Table 42 it can be seen that consultant involvement was highest during the day (39.6% of cases presenting during the day) and fell over the evening and into the night (11.5% of cases presenting during night). The trend for staff in training involvement was in the opposite direction. Notably SHOs were the first reviewer/team leader in 20.4% (23/113) of cases at night.

While this pattern of reduced consultant involvement and increased junior staff involvement during the evenings and night is not new data, it is concerning since trauma often presents out of hours when the hospital is least well staffed to deal with these challenges. It is clear that patients presenting in the evenings and nights were, in the view of the advisors, being subjected to a lesser standard of care than during the daytime.

Table 42. Time of day by grade of reviewer

	Day (08.00-17.59)		Evening (18.00-23.59)		Night (00.00-07.59)	
Grade	**Number of patients**		**Number of patients**		**Number of patients**	
		%		%		%
Consultant	82	39.6	40	27.8	13	11.5
NCCG	56	27.1	45	31.3	24	21.2
SpR 3+	28	13.5	31	21.5	34	30.1
SpR 1/2	17	8.2	17	11.8	15	13.3
SHO	22	10.6	9	6.3	23	20.4
Nurse	1	<1	1	<1	1	<1
Other	1	<1	1	<1	3	2.7
Total	**207**		**144**		**113**	

Relationship between grade of reviewer and quality of care

As stated previously, the experience of the staff making the initial assessment and leading the trauma team is one of the factors that may impact on patient outcome. One question that was asked of the advisors during the peer review process was 'was the initial response in hospital appropriate?'.

It was possible to look at the relationship between the advisors' opinion on appropriateness of initial response and the grade of initial reviewer/team leader in 477/795 cases. In 318 cases, poor documentation of clinicians' grades prevented this analysis. Overall 51 of the 477 (10.7%) cases that could be assessed were considered to have an inappropriate response. When these data were disaggregated by grade of first reviewer a clearer picture emerged and the percentage of inappropriate responses rose from 3.1% (5/159) when consultants were the first reviewer to 23.5% (16/68) when SHOs were the first reviewer (Table 43).

Table 43. Appropriate response by grade of reviewer (advisors' view)

	Appropriate response				
Grade of first reviewer	**Yes**		**No**		**Total**
		%		**%**	
Consultant	154	96.9	5	3.1	159
NCCG	16	84.2	3	15.8	19
SpR	204	88.3	27	11.7	231
SHO	52	76.5	16	23.5	68
Total	**426**		**51**		**477**

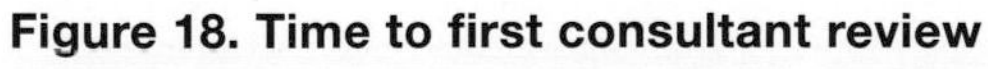

Figure 18. Time to first consultant review

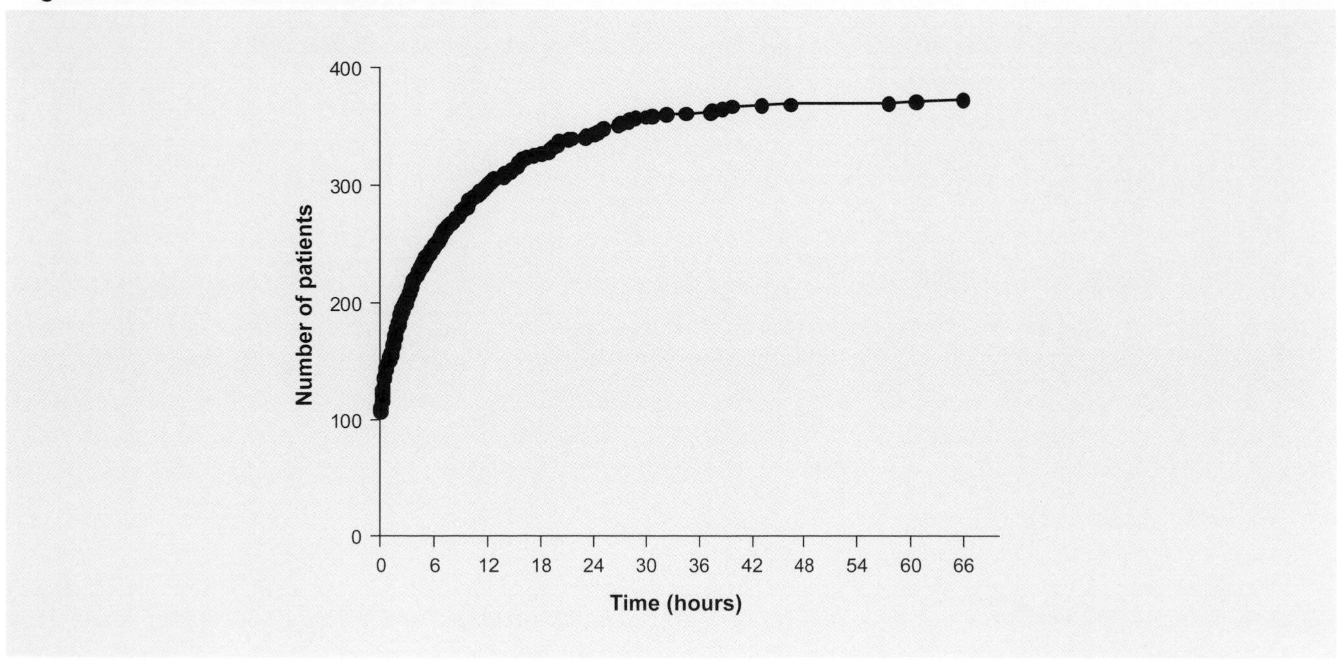

These data provide a clear association between grade of first reviewer and the advisors' assessments of appropriateness of response.

Table 44. Time to first consultant review

	Number of patients	%
On arrival	108	29.0
> 0 ≤ 30 minutes	34	9.1
> 30 minutes ≤ 1 hour	12	3.2
> 1 hour ≤ 6 hours	96	25.7
> 6 hours ≤ 12 hours	53	14.2
> 12 hours	70	18.8
Subtotal	**373**	
Insufficient data	422	
Total	**795**	

As can be seen from Figure 18 and Table 44, a substantial proportion (18.8%) of patients had not been reviewed by a consultant within 12 hours of arrival to hospital. A number of patients had still not been seen within 24 hours of arrival. In addition, it is worth reiterating that 176/513 patients (34.3%; data from the A&E clinician questionnaire) were not seen by a consultant in the emergency department. The time to first consultant review could only be calculated for 373/795 (47%) cases. Poor documentation of review times and grade of reviewer are large contributory factors to this.

Prompt review by consultant staff would appear to be a sensible aim. The influence of consultant staff is most likely to be seen in the domain of the decision-making process. Put more simply, consultants should have the training, ability and seniority to ensure that the correct actions are undertaken in a prompt and efficient manner, thereby improving the patient care process. It was recently shown in a study of severely injured patients[5] that consultant presence in the emergency department reduced the mean time to operating theatre in these patients: (43.8 minutes (+/-20.1) when a consultant was present and 109.4 minutes (+/-10.7) when a consultant was not present, $p<0.05$). In addition there were no missed injuries, delays to the operating theatre, or inappropriate workups when a consultant was present. It is, therefore, a concern that a number of severely injured patients within this study experienced significant delays before consultant involvement. Furthermore, the high percentage of inappropriate initial responses when consultants were not immediately involved (Table 41) supports this view.

Primary survey and overall assessment

Primary survey

In 88.8% (706/795) of cases a primary survey was documented on arrival in the emergency department (Table 45). In the opinion of the advisors this primary survey was performed sufficiently early enough in 680/706 (96.3%) cases, not sufficiently early enough in 26 cases (3.7%) and there was insufficient data to comment in 89 cases (Table 46).

Table 45. Documentation of a primary survey

	Number of patients	%
Yes	706	88.8
No	89	11.2
Total	**795**	

Table 46. Timeliness of a primary survey

	Number of patients	%
Yes	680	96.3
No	26	3.7
Subtotal	**706**	
Insufficient data	89	
Total	**795**	

Despite the widespread adoption of the ATLS system no primary survey was documented in 11.2% (89/795) of cases. Immediate management of life-threatening emergencies and identification of major injuries is a key to good outcomes for severely injured patients and it is difficult to see how this can reliably happen in the absence of a primary survey.

Appropriateness of initial response

The advisors were asked to assess the initial response to the trauma patient. Table 47 shows that of the 699 cases that could be assessed, 94 (13.4%) were graded as having an inappropriate initial response. In a further 96/795 cases, there was insufficient data to comment.

Table 47. Appropriateness of initial response

	Number of patients	%
Yes	605	86.6
No	94	13.4
Subtotal	**699**	
Insufficient data	96	
Total	**795**	

Overall assessment and appropriateness of initial response

Part of the advisors' role was to come to an overall assessment of each case using the grading system described in the method section. Table 48 shows how the patients classified as having an inappropriate initial response were graded (94/699 from Table 47).

Table 48. Overall assessment in patients with inappropriate initial response

	Number of patients	%
Good practice	8	8.5
Room for improvement clinical	28	29.8
Room for improvement organisational	17	18.1
Room for improvement clinical and organisational	21	22.3
Less than satisfactory	17	18.1
Insufficient data	3	3.2
Total	**94**	

Only a small number of the cases (8/94) were graded as good practice. Additionally, in the view of the advisors, 17 patients received less than satisfactory care. The above reflects the importance of the initial response, in terms of clinical decision-making and overall care for the severely injured patient.

Key findings

A pre-alert from the ambulance crew to the receiving emergency department was documented for only 50.1% of patients in this study.

One in five hospitals admitting severely injured patients did not have a formal trauma team.

When a pre-alert was made to the receiving emergency department, there was no trauma response in one in four cases.

A trauma team response was documented for only 59.7% of patients in this study.

A consultant was the team leader/ first reviewer in only 169/419 (40.3%) of cases.

Advisors felt that the patient's initial management was inappropriate in 23.5% of cases where an SHO was the team leader/ first reviewer compared to 3.1% of cases where a consultant was the team leader/ first reviewer.

If no trauma response was activated, then it was more likely that an SHO was the first reviewer or team leader for the severely injured patient.

176/419 (42%) patients were not seen by a consultant in the emergency department.

89/795 (11.2%) patients did not have a primary survey documented in their casenotes.

The initial management of the patient was thought to be inappropriate in 94/699 cases (13.4%).

Recommendations

Ambulance trusts and emergency departments should have clear guidelines for the use of pre-alerts in the severely injured patient population. The ambulance crew should be able to speak directly to clinical staff in the receiving emergency department to ensure an appropriate clinical response is available immediately. *(Ambulance trusts and emergency departments)*

Trusts should ensure that a trauma team is available 24 hours a day, seven days a week. This is an essential part of an organised trauma response system. *(Hospital trusts)*

Hospital and ambulance trusts should ensure there are agreed explicit criteria for issuing a pre-alert activation of the trauma team. *(Hospital and ambulance trusts)*

A consultant must be the team leader for the management of the severely injured patient. There should be no reason for this not to happen during the normal working week. Trusts and consultants should work together to provide job plans that will lead to better consultant presence in the emergency department at all times to provide more uniform consultant leadership for all severely injured patients. *(Hospital trusts and clinical directors)*

All patients should have a primary survey performed and clearly documented on admission to the emergency department. *(Emergency medicine physicians)*

Standardised documentation for the trauma patient should be developed. This will improve patient care and multidisciplinary communication. In addition, comparative audit will be facilitated. *(RCS and College of Emergency Medicine)*

As previously recommended, a consultant must be the team leader for the management of the severely injured patient. However, it is appreciated that this will not be achievable immediately. In the absence of this standard all severely injured patients should be reviewed by a consultant as soon as possible; ideally this should be within four hours of arrival at hospital, but must be within 12 hours of arrival. *(Hospital trusts)*

References

1. The Royal College of Surgeons of England and the British Orthopaedic Society. *Better Care for the Severely Injured.* 2000

2. Kazemi AR, Nayeem N. *The existence and composition of trauma teams in the UK.* Injury 1997; 28:119-21

3. Brooks A, Williams J, Butcher W, Ryan J. *General Surgeons and Trauma. A questionnaire survey of General Surgeons training in ATLS and involvement in the trauma team.* Injury 2003; 34(7):484-6

4. Yates DW, Woodford M, Hollis S. *Preliminary analysis of the care of injured patients in 33 British hospitals: first report of the United Kingdom major trauma outcome study.* BMJ 1992; 305(6856):737-40

5. Porter JM, Ursic C. *Trauma attending in the resuscitation room: does it affect outcome?* Am Surg 2001; 67(7):611-4

CHAPTER 6 - Airway and breathing

Introduction

Adequate oxygenation of the tissues is critical to survival after trauma, and the maintenance of adequate levels of oxygen in the blood stream is a paramount objective in the management of severe trauma. Tissue hypoxia may occur as a result of multiple injuries, haemorrhage or depressed respiration and it may occur acutely or insidiously. A leading, but rapidly reversible, life-threatening cause of insufficient oxygenation is obstruction of the airway. Therefore, the reversal of an obstructed airway is regarded as fundamental in any approach to managing the severely injured patient.

Airway management is therefore one of the key components of emergency care. The primary objective is to recognise an obstructed or potentially obstructed airway, to clear the obstruction and keep the airway patent. No medical emergency, short of complete cardiopulmonary arrest, is more immediately life-threatening than the loss of an adequate airway. Failure to manage airway patency and ventilation adequately has been identified as a major cause of preventable death in trauma[1-4].

Many studies highlight the preventable mortality and morbidity that occur following major trauma[5, 6]. Airway problems and hypovolaemia are very often the causes. The advanced trauma life support (ATLS) system of trauma care stresses the importance of recognition of airway and ventilation problems. The value of early senior experienced anaesthetic involvement cannot be over-stated. The anaesthetist should be a key member of the resuscitation trauma team, and not simply called when serious problems have already developed.

Results

Airway and ventilation in hospital

Table 49 shows the airway status on arrival at the emergency department and the 72 hour mortality for each group of patients. As can be seen, 85/676 (12.6%) of patients arrive at hospital with either a partially or completely obstructed airway and these groups had a much higher mortality rate although from this dataset, causality cannot be assumed.

Table 49. Airway status on arrival at hospital

	Alive	Deceased	Total	% Mortality
Clear	526	65	**591**	11.0
Noisy	27	13	**40**	32.5
Blocked	28	17	**45**	37.8
Subtotal	**581**	**95**	**676**	
Not recorded	97	22	**119**	18.5
Total	**678**	**117**	**795**	

The provision of an adequate airway by intubation of the trachea is often required to facilitate the management of the severely injured patient. Table 50 shows that 74 patients were intubated before arrival at hospital, 11 patients had attempted but failed intubation and 362 patients were intubated after arrival at hospital. Table 50 also shows mortality rates at 72 hours after injury. It can be seen that the group that was intubated prehospital had a higher mortality than the group intubated in hospital. This is in line with previous literature[7] although a causal relationship cannot be determined from this dataset.

There are issues with prehospital and hospital airway management. In the prehospital chapter concerns were raised about the delays on scene whilst attempting to secure an airway. Despite the prehospital care, 12.6% of patients arrived at hospital with a partially or completely obstructed airway. This raises questions about what forms of airway provision should be used in the prehospital phase, what skills the prehospital staff need to possess and what background these practitioners should come from (paramedical, medical).

Table 50. Intubation status and mortality

	Alive	Deceased	Total	% Mortality
Prehospital	45	29	**74**	39.2
Failed attempt (prehospital)	3	8	**11**	72.7
Hospital	290	72	**362**	19.9
Subtotal	**338**	**109**	**447**	
No evidence	340	8	**348**	2.3
Total	**678**	**117**	**795**	

Table 51. Grade of clinician involved with intubation

	Number of patients	%
Consultant	22	15.8
SpR	95	68.3
SHO	22	15.8
Subtotal	**139**	
Not recorded	223	
Total	**362**	

Table 52. Specialty of clinician involved with intubation

	Number of patients	%
Anaesthetics	203	88.3
Critical care medicine	20	8.7
Emergency medicine	7	3.0
Subtotal	**230**	
Not recorded	132	
Total	**362**	

Tables 51 and 52 show data relevant to the personnel involved in, and the timing of, tracheal intubation. Data on grade of medical staff involved was poorly documented and not available in 223/362 cases. Anaesthetists were responsible for the majority of this activity (203/230 cases – 88.3%). There was evidence for use of rapid sequence induction in 237/362 (65.5%) patients intubated in hospital.

In a substantial number of cases the grade and/or specialty were not recorded. Where data were available it is clear that many patients were intubated on arrival at hospital or very shortly after. This, combined with the 12.6% of patients who arrived at hospital with an obstructed or partially obstructed airway, raises concerns over the adequacy of prehospital airway management under the current system of prehospital care, which is largely provided by paramedic staff who are not trained to use drugs to facilitate tracheal intubation.

Table 53. Time of intubation (minutes)

	Number of patients	%
On arrival	54	22.2
0 ≥ 10	31	12.8
> 10 ≤ 20	21	8.6
> 20 ≤ 30	25	10.3
> 30 ≤ 40	10	4.1
> 40 ≤ 50	10	4.1
> 50 ≤ 60	7	2.9
> 60	85	35.0
Subtotal	**243**	
Not recorded	119	
Total	**362**	

Figure 19. First hospital respiration rate

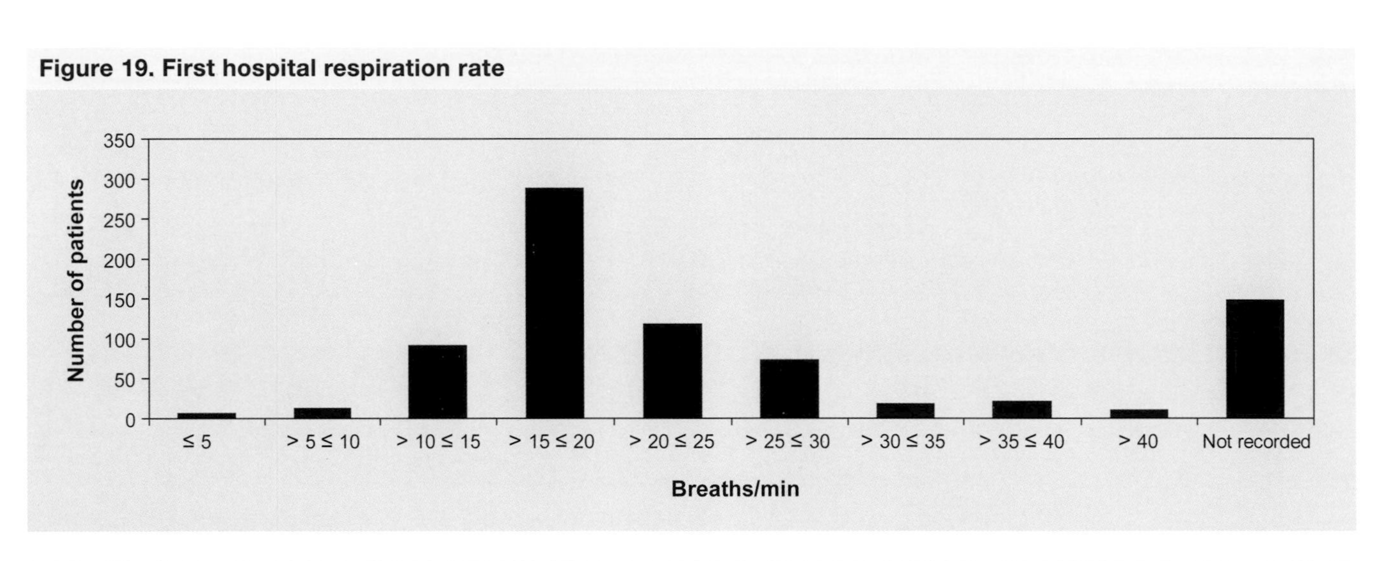

Figure 20. First hospital SpO_2

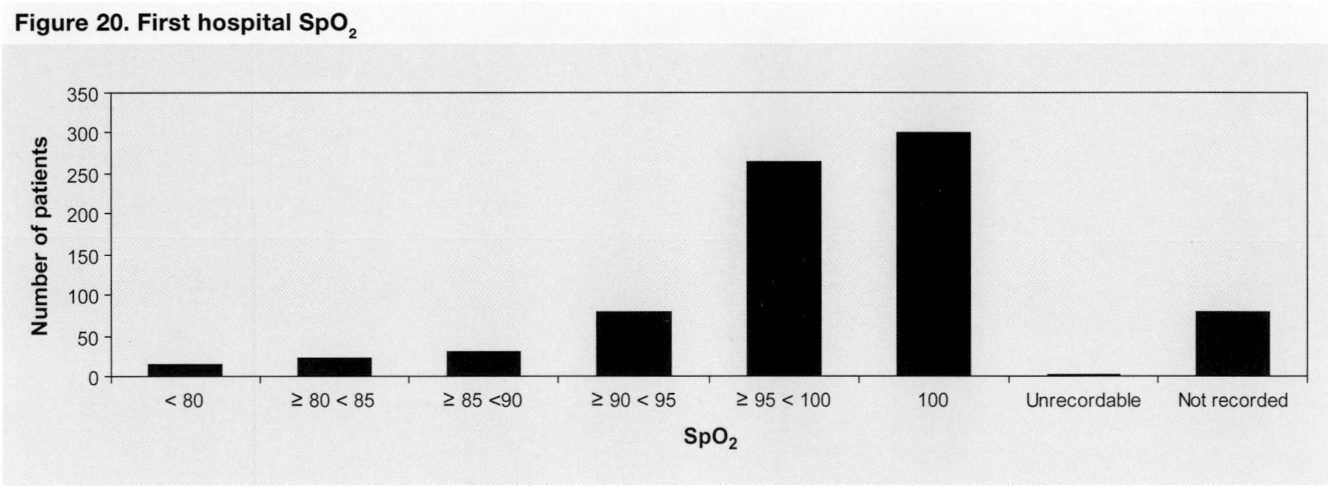

Figure 19 shows the initial respiratory rate on admission to the emergency department. Many patients had an abnormal respiratory rate reflecting their underlying injuries. Respiratory rate is a very sensitive indicator of critical illness and progression of disease. This parameter was not recorded in 149 of 795 cases (18.7%). This lack of respiratory rate monitoring has been found in other studies of severely ill patients[8] and despite recommendations for more use of this measurement; the situation has changed little in this study. The SpO_2 was recorded in all but 81/795 (10.2%) cases on admission (Figure 20).

Figures 21, 22 and 23 show data from the first arterial blood gas (ABG) analysis after admission to the emergency department. A large number 334/795 (42%) of patients did not have arterial blood gas analysis, which is surprising in the setting of severe trauma. Of those who did have arterial blood gas analysis, it can be seen that there is extreme physiological derangement in a substantial number.

Figure 21. First ABG pH measurements

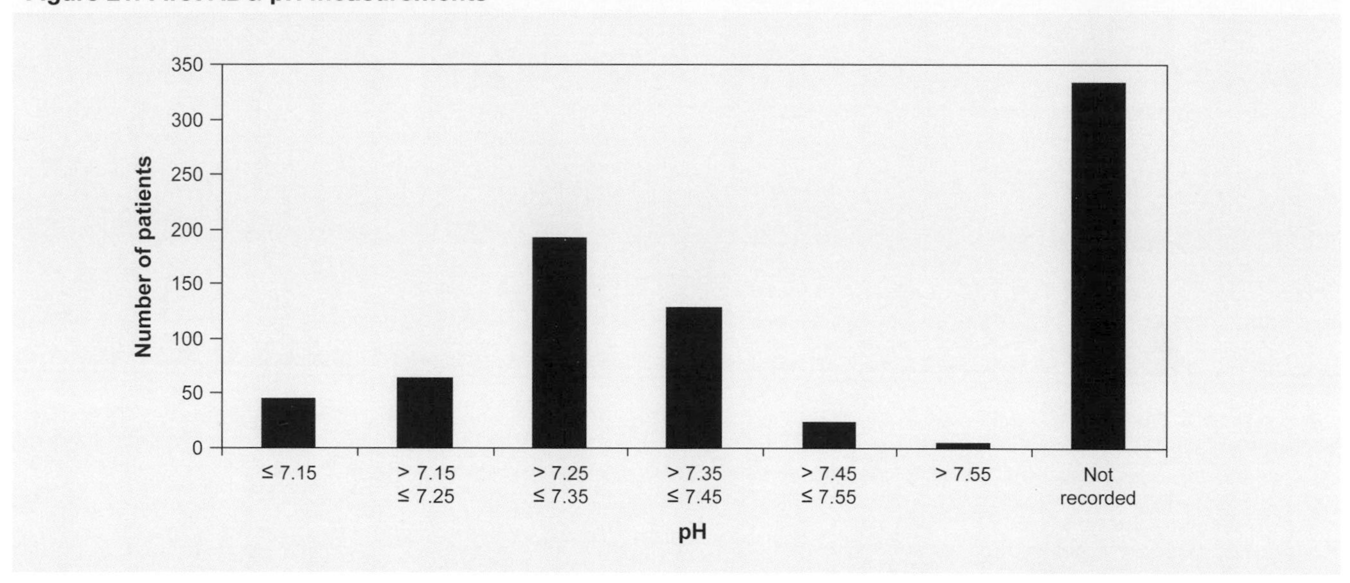

Figure 22. First ABG PaO_2 measurements

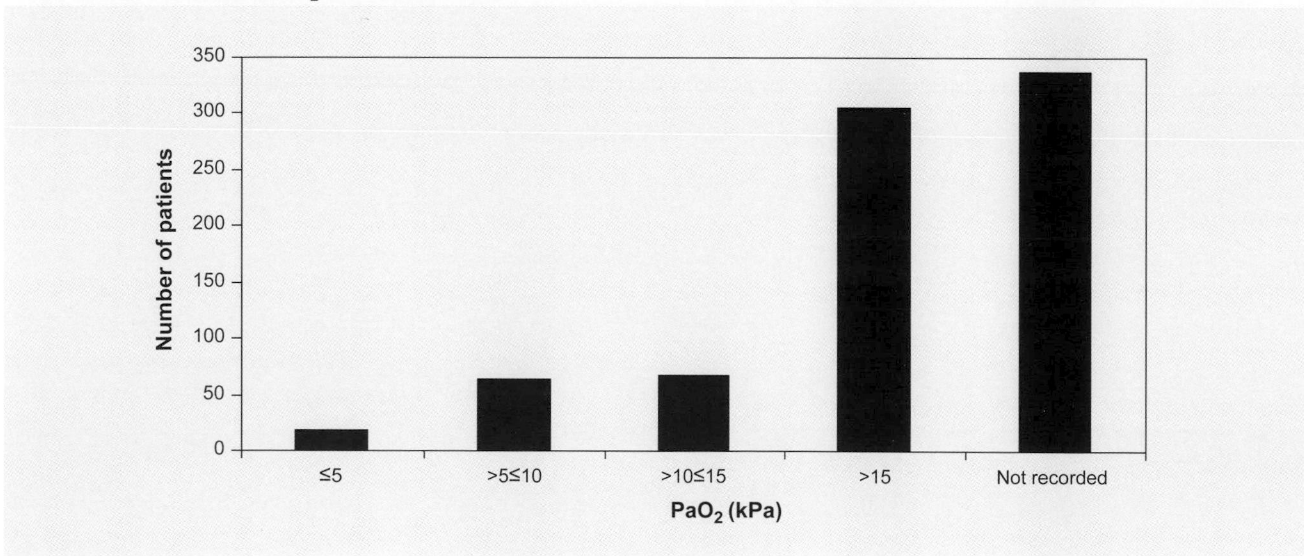

Figure 23. First ABG $PaCO_2$ measurements

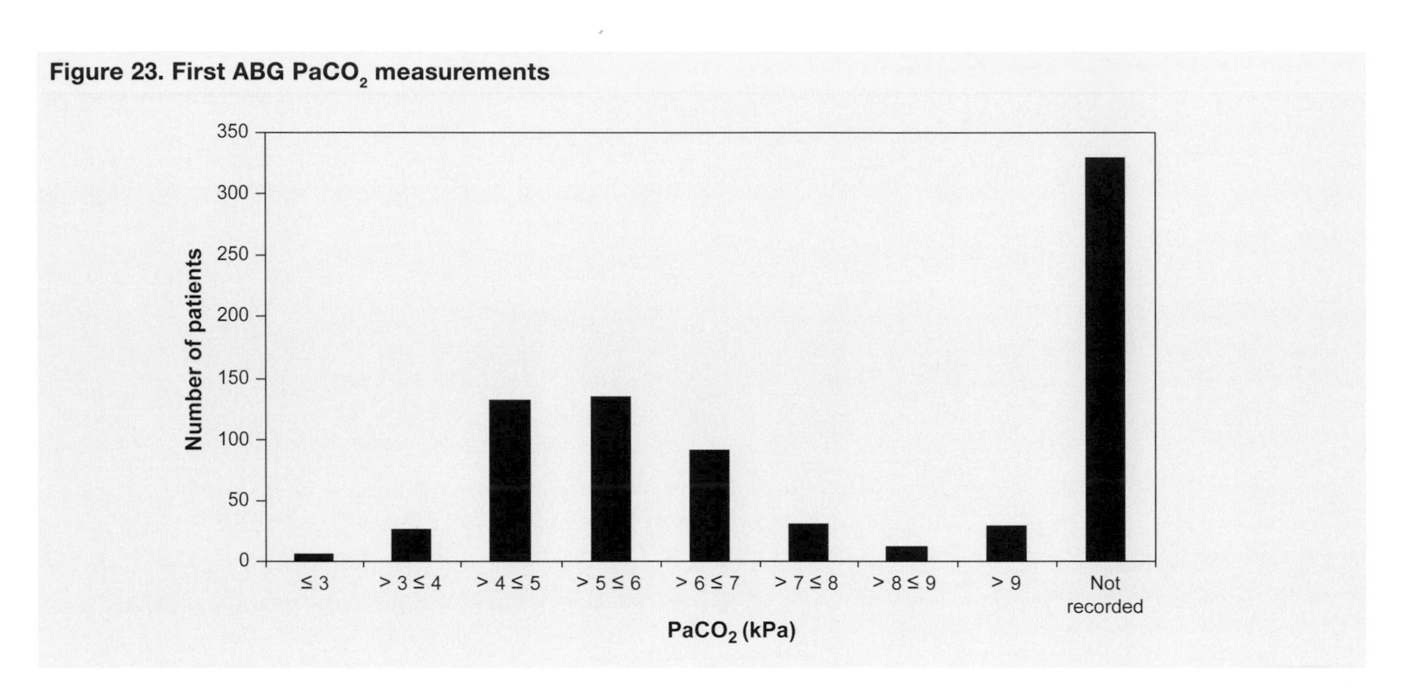

One of the challenges in the trauma patient can be provision of an adequate airway[9] and tracheal intubation is frequently a much more difficult procedure in the trauma patient[10]. Table 54 shows that in 56/753 (7.4%) cases, the advisors saw evidence of difficulty in obtaining an adequate airway. In 42 cases it was not possible to assess this. Of interest was whether this was associated with the grade or experience of personnel involved. Unfortunately, the information on the personnel involved was so poorly documented, that no comment can be made on this relationship.

Table 54. Evidence of difficulty in obtaining an airway

	Number of patients	%
Yes	56	7.4
No	697	92.6
Subtotal	**753**	
Insufficient data	42	
Total	**795**	

The group of patients who are difficult to intubate may have different injuries, or a greater severity of injury, compared to the group in whom there was no difficulty with intubation. The mortality rate at 72 hours in the group of patients with airway difficulty was 25% (14/56) compared with 13.6% (95/697) in the non-difficult group. However, it is not clear if there was any direct causal relationship between the difficulty with airway provision and mortality.

Advisors were asked to make an overall assessment of the management of the airway and breathing. From Table 55 it can be seen that this was considered unsatisfactory in 52/741 cases (7%) where the data could be assessed.

Table 55. Satisfactory airway management

	Number of patients	%
Yes	689	93.0
No	52	7.0
Subtotal	**741**	
Insufficient data	54	
Total	**795**	

Cervical spine management

The National Institute for Health and Clinical Excellence (NICE) guidance on management of head injuries[11] recognises the problems of cervical spine imaging in some circumstances and states that:

> "The current initial investigation of choice for the detection of injuries to the cervical spine is the plain radiograph. Three views should be obtained and be of sufficient quality for reliable interpretation. However, in certain circumstances CT is preferred.
>
> **GCS below 13 on initial assessment,**
>
> **has been intubated,**
>
> **plain film series is technically inadequate (for example, desired view unavailable), suspicious or definitely abnormal,**
>
> **continued clinical suspicion of injury despite a normal x-ray,**
>
> **the patient is being scanned for multi-region trauma".**

All severely injured patients who undergo CT imaging of the head, or other body parts, should have CT imaging of the cervical spine performed at the same time.

Table 56. Prehospital spine immobilisation

	Number of patients	%
Cervical spine	32	9.6
Whole spine	45	13.6
Cervical spine & whole spine	255	76.8
Subtotal	**332**	
Neither documented	172	
Total	**504**	

Table 56 shows data on what protection was given to the cervical spine, and whole spine, in the prehospital phase (data from PRF).

Of the 172 patients with no cervical spine immobilisation documented in the prehospital phase 69 had cervical spine immobilisation on admission to the emergency department (40.1%).

Table 57 shows the advisors' assessment of measures to control the cervical spine. Overall there was concern that in 55/660 (8.3%) cases where it could be assessed the cervical spine was not adequately managed. In 135 cases there was insufficient data for the advisors to make an assessment.

Table 57. Appropriate control of cervical spine (advisors' opinion)

	Yes	No	Subtotal	Insufficient data	Total
Prehospital	332	6	**338**	35	**373**
In hospital	166	15	**181**	29	**210**
Subtotal	**498**	**21**	**519**	**64**	**583**
Not recorded	107	34	**141**	71	**212**
Total	**605**	**55**	**660**	**135**	**795**

Table 58 shows reasons for advisors' concerns.

Table 58. Reasons for advisors' concerns with regard to inappropriate control of cervical spine	
No evidence of protection	22
Delay in protection	5
Not appropriately cleared	11
Needed imaging	3
Unable to fit collar	4
Other	10
Total	**55**

Imaging and clearance of the cervical spine was often commented on during the peer review process. There were frequent problems with adequate imaging of the cervical spine in unconscious patients. There were often multiple attempts at plain x-rays of the cervical spine, even in those patients who were undergoing CT scanning of another body part. Reluctance to provide CT imaging of the cervical spine at the same time as head CT scan was commonly encountered.

Case study 1

A young patient was admitted following a motor vehicle crash. Initial Glasgow Coma Score was 5 and the right pupil was fixed and dilated. The patient was transferred for a CT head scan which showed some cerebral contusions and swelling but no lesion requiring neurosurgical intervention. Given the mechanism of injury there was concern that the cervical spine may also have been damaged. No CT of the cervical spine was performed; instead the patient was transferred back to the emergency department to have plain x-rays of the cervical spine. Despite several attempts, plain x-rays provided inadequate views of the whole cervical spine and the patient was then transferred back to the CT scanner for CT imaging of the cervical spine.

The clinical scenario in Case study 1 was not uncommon.

Key findings

One in eight patients arrived at hospital with either a partially or completely obstructed airway.

Prehospital intubation failed on 11/85 attempts (12.9%).

131 patients were intubated either on admission or within the first 30 minutes after admission to hospital.

Data on grade of medical staff performing tracheal intubation was poorly documented and not available in 223/362 cases (61.6%).

Management of the airway was considered unsatisfactory in 52/741 cases (7%).

The management of the potentially unstable spine was considered unsatisfactory in 55/660 cases (8.3%).

Recommendations

The current structure of prehospital management is insufficient to meet the needs of the severely injured patient. There is a high incidence of failed intubation and a high incidence of patients arriving at hospital with a partially or completely obstructed airway. Change is urgently required to provide a system that reliably provides a clear airway with good oxygenation and control of ventilation. This may be through the provision of personnel with the ability to provide anaesthesia and intubation in the prehospital phase or the use of alternative airway devices. *(Ambulance trusts)*

CT scanning of the cervical spine should be performed in adult patients who have any of the following features:

- GCS below 13 on initial assessment
- has been intubated
- is being scanned for multi-region trauma

(Radiology heads)

References

1. Gorman DF, Teanby DN, Sinha MP, Wotherspoon J, Boot DA, Molokhia A. *Preventable deaths among major trauma patients in Mersey Region, North Wales and the Isle of Man.* Injury 1996; 27:189–92

2. Esposito TJ, Sanddal ND, Dean JM, Hansen JD, Reynolds SA, Battan K. *Analysis of preventable pediatric trauma deaths and inappropriate trauma care in Montana.* The Journal of Trauma 1999; 47:243–51

3. Papadopoulos IN, Bukis D, Karalas E, Katsaragakis S, Stergiopoulos S, Peros G, Androulakis G. *Preventable prehospital trauma deaths in a Hellenic urban health region: an audit of prehospital trauma care.* The Journal of Trauma 1996; 41:864–9

4. Hussain LM, Redmond AD. *Are prehospital deaths from accidental injury preventable?* BMJ 1994; 23:1077–80

5. Cales RH, Trunkey DD. *Preventable trauma deaths.* JAMA 1985; 254: 1059-63

6. Anderson ID, Woodford M, Donbal FT, Irving M. *Retrospective Study of 1000 Deaths from Injury in England and Wales.* BMJ 1989; 296:1305-8

7. Lockey D, Davies G, Coats T. *Survival of trauma patients who have prehospital tracheal intubation without anaesthesia or muscle relaxants: observational study.* BMJ 2001;323:141

8. *An Acute Problem?* National Confidential Enquiry into Patient Outcome and Death. 2005. *http://www.ncepod.org.uk*

9. Boegtz MS, Katz JA. *Airway management of the trauma patient.* Semin Anaes 1985; 4:114-23

10. Dunham CM, Barraco RD, Clark DE, Daley BJ, Davis FE 3rd, Gibbs MA, Knuth T, Letarte PB, Luchette FA, Omert L, Weireter LJ, Wiles CE 3rd; EAST Practice Management Guidelines Work Group. *Guidelines for emergency tracheal intubation immediately after traumatic injury.* J Trauma 2003; 55:162-197

11. National Institute for Health and Clinical Excellence. Draft NICE head injury guidance 2007 – *http://guidance.nice.org.uk/page.aspx?o=267085&c=91522*

CHAPTER 7 - Management of circulation

Introduction

The importance of haemorrhage control after injury is crucial. Best published evidence suggests that 30-40% of early trauma deaths are directly attributable to haemorrhage[1,2]. The American College of Surgeons Committee on Trauma Multiple Outcome Study has estimated that 62% of all in-hospital trauma deaths occur within the first four hours, of which haemorrhage is either the primary cause or a major contributing factor[3]. Not only does haemorrhage contribute directly to early mortality, but blood loss leading to hypotension is a major factor in the development of secondary brain injury[4,5] as well as contributing significantly to late trauma deaths from multi-organ failure[6,7].

Shock is a condition of inadequate end-organ perfusion. In the severely injured patient, shock may be multifactorial, but haemorrhage is the leading aetiology. In the shocked polytrauma patient, the physiologic and metabolic reserve can quickly become exhausted, leading to decompensation and a deadly triad of hypothermia, coagulopathy and acidosis, all of which are independent prognostic indicators of outcome[8-13]. Treatment of these patients is aimed at preventing or reversing this metabolic derangement by recognising firstly that haemorrhage exists (preferentially before decompensation), followed by timely intervention to arrest the bleeding and restore circulating volume, and hence oxygenation, to the tissues. Such timely management is associated with improved patient outcomes[14,15].

The management of haemorrhage should begin in the prehospital field and continue right through the hospital system in a continuous process of assessment, treatment and reassessment in a timely, co-ordinated fashion. Modern, dedicated trauma systems and major trauma centres have developed out of a need for rapid transportation, assessment and treatment of the bleeding patient. Such dedicated shock-trauma systems are associated with shorter prehospital times[16-18], shorter throughput times to definitive care at an appropriate facility[19,20] and better outcomes for the severely injured patient[16, 21-24]. Nevertheless, the majority of preventable deaths after injury occur from unrecognised and hence untreated haemorrhage, particularly within the abdominal cavity[25-28] making it perhaps the single most important reversible cause of death in the trauma population.

Defining the point at which a patient becomes 'shocked' is difficult as bleeding patients are often in a state of dynamic physiologic flux. However, recognition of ongoing bleeding is the first step in management. The Advanced Trauma Life Support (ATLS) course has become a well-recognised and accepted paradigm in the initial management of the bleeding patient. Although the optimum end points for effective resuscitation are less clear clinically[29,30], current practice in the acute assessment of the injured patient is based on a dictum of readily available and measurable parameters such as blood pressure, pulse rate, respiratory rate, capillary refill, oxygen saturations and Glasgow Coma Score. This has formed the basis for the format of questions in the management of circulation after injury for this NCEPOD study. These are simple bedside assessments which may be repeated, and aim to recognise the bleeding patient early. In the physiologically normal, stable patient who has not decompensated, time allows for more detailed diagnostic workup for occult bleeding and organ injury. Simple, rapidly performed tests should also be performed early in management that may reflect both regional and global hypoperfusion including; pH, lactate, base deficit and bicarbonate levels[31-36].

The modern approach to the management of haemorrhage after injury has evolved greatly in the two decades with the advent of better evidence based practice. Older diagnostic tests, such as diagnostic peritoneal lavage (DPL) have now been largely superseded by other imaging techniques such as bedside ultrasound (focussed abdominal sonography for trauma (FAST))[37-39] and more judicious use of CT scanning for the physiological normal and stable patient. In many ways, CT scanning is the ideal non-invasive test as long as the patient's condition allows. As a result many injuries can now be safely managed conservatively or non-operatively[40,41]. Advances in radiology have allowed a greater proportion of bleeding patients to undergo successful angioembolisation of bleeding arterial vessels, especially for injuries that are traditionally difficult to manage operatively or are associated with a high mortality[42,43].

Other important standards of care have now become commonplace for the exsanguinating trauma patient subgroup. These approaches, which are almost counterintuitive to classical surgical dogma, include hypotensive resuscitation and damage control surgery. These concepts place a much greater emphasis on permissive blood pressure control at a subnormal but survivable level, followed by rapid, intraoperative control of haemorrhage in a staged fashion and less on diagnostic workup and definitive treatment of injuries during the early stages of treatment. Both concepts have been associated with higher survival rates for the exsanguinating subgroup of injured patients[44-46].

Despite the modern approach to the bleeding patient, there is still one concept that has remained unchanged. Blood is a precious commodity and early haemorrhage control, whether it occurs naturally or after iatrogenic intervention such as angioembolisation or intraoperatively by a surgeon, is still paramount in achieving good patient outcomes. Thus, effective and timely haemorrhage recognition and control may be the single most important step in the emergency management of the severely injured patient.

Results

Initial haemodynamic assessment

The casenotes available identified that assessment of pulse, blood pressure, capillary refill and temperature were measured on arrival at hospital in 95.4%, 95.7%, 31.6% and 53.2% of cases respectively (Figure 24).

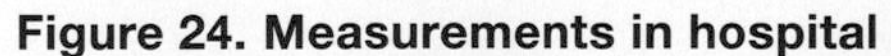

Figure 24. Measurements in hospital

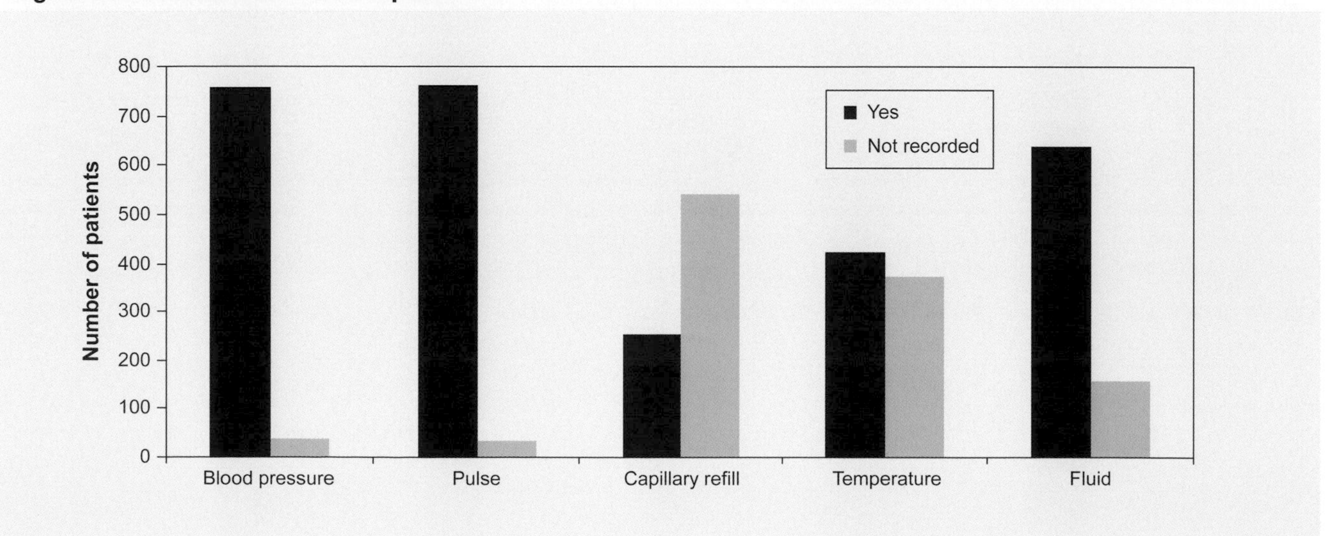

Figure 25. Appropriate fluid resuscitation to the degree of shock

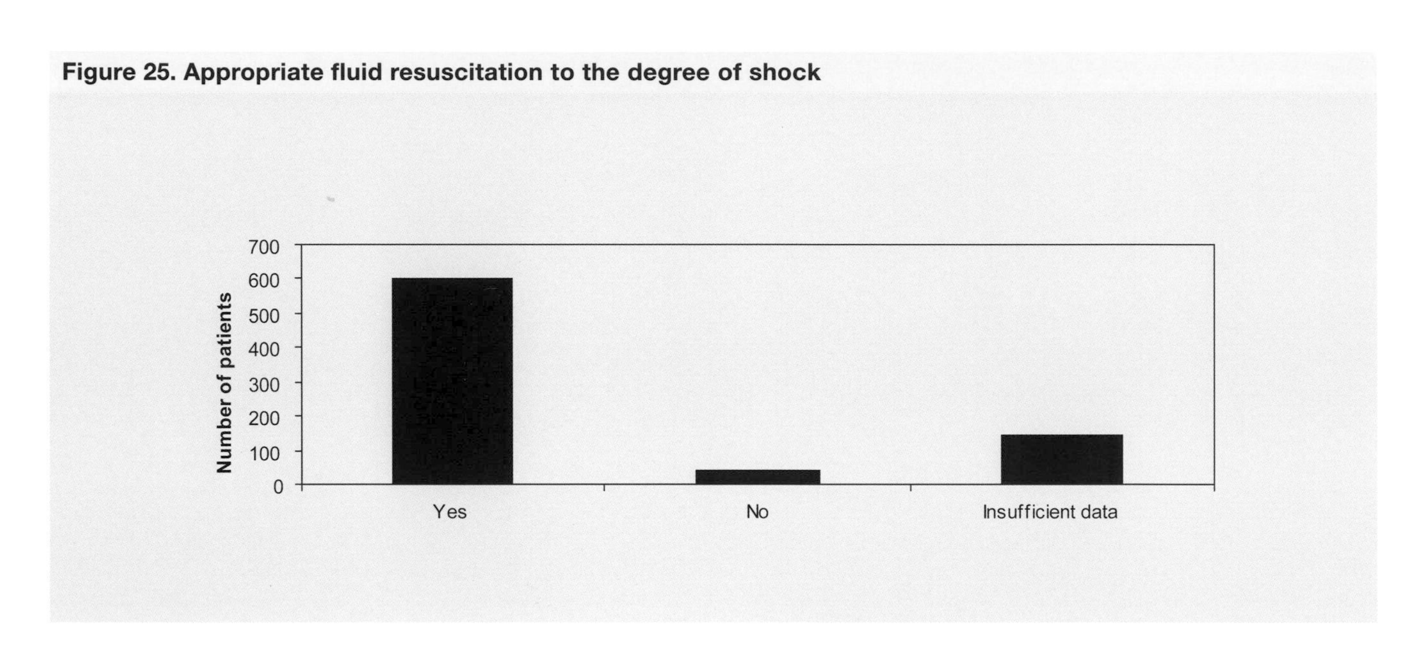

Fluid therapy

Fluids were administered to 638/795 (80.3%) patients.

Appropriateness of fluid therapy

It was assessed by the advisors that fluid resuscitation was appropriate in 93.2% (602/646) of patients and inappropriate in 44/646 cases (6.8%).

In 16 cases it was considered that there was very aggressive fluid therapy and that too much crystalloid was given. In five cases it was considered that blood, rather than continued crystalloid, should have been transfused, as there was very significant haemorrhage. In 21 cases it was considered that insufficient fluid was given.

Case study 2

A young back seat passenger was involved in a high-speed road traffic collision. Glasgow Coma Score was 14 on admission. A CT head scan excluded significant head injury. Haemoglobin level fell from 12 to 6 over three hours. The eventual injuries identified were: pelvic fracture; splenic and renal lacerations; and mediastinal haematoma. There was only one measurement of blood pressure in the first hour of admission and no IV access. When the blood loss was recognised, the patient was over transfused with six litres of crystalloid and three units of blood.

Figure 26. CT scan of the chest, abdomen or pelvis performed

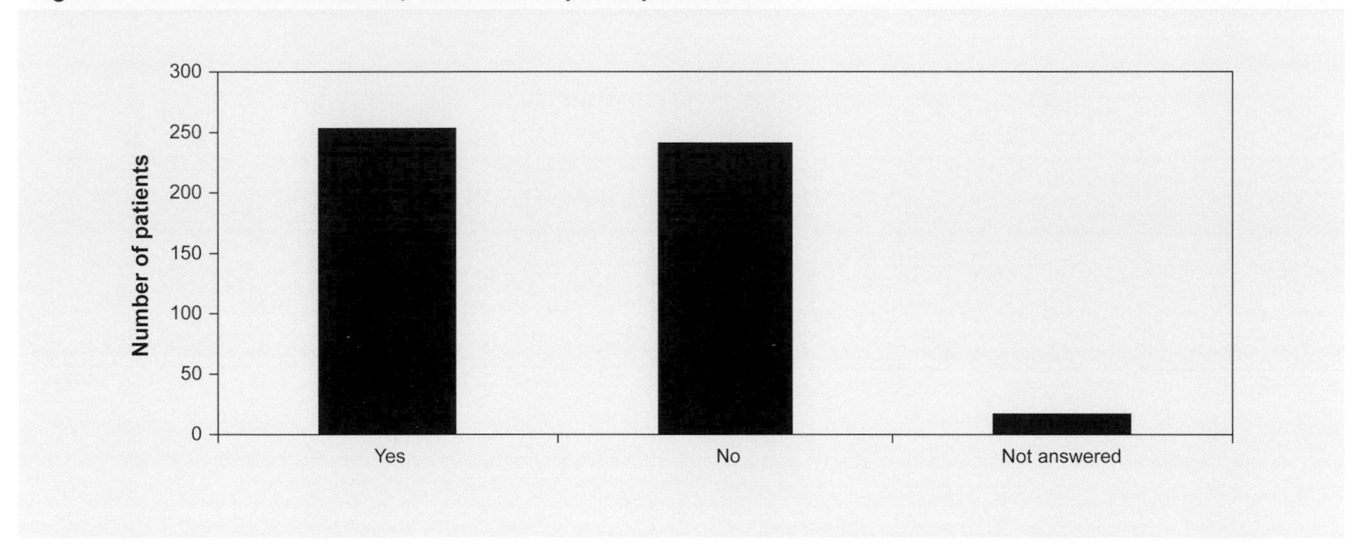

Investigation of haemorrhage

It is often the case that an experienced trauma surgeon will identify patients who need an immediate trauma laparotomy simply by the nature of the trauma and their failure to respond to fluid therapy. In these cases further investigation may be unnecessary and delay the time to definitive care, which is associated with poorer outcomes.

Some patients will require further investigation and options include DPL, FAST or CT scanning. The availability of these options is described in the organisational chapter. Whilst the use of DPL is falling as a consequence of better access to more sophisticated imaging, only one in three emergency departments had access to FAST.

Use of investigations

Clinicians completing the A&E questionnaire indicated that 254/495 (51.3%) patients had a CT scan of the chest and/or abdomen and/or pelvis for the assessment of injuries and potential haemorrhage. For 18 patients this question was not answered (Figure 26).

For the large majority of patients (185/241; 76.8%) the reason given for not scanning the chest, abdomen or pelvis was because it was not clinically indicated. However, 22 patients did not have a CT scan as they were considered too unstable to be transferred to the CT scanner. For a further three patients it was indicated that they were taken straight to theatre. There was one case where a scan could not be performed as the CT scanner was broken.

The percentage of patients requiring CT for investigation for haemorrhage was found to be higher on assessment of the casenotes (483/795; 60.8%) compared to that reported in the A&E questionnaire. This was simply because of the difference in the returned documentation (513 A&E questionnaires v 795 sets of casenotes), there were no cases for which a discrepancy was found between the casenotes and A&E questionnaire. Three hundred and ninety three patients had a CT alone and 90 patients had a CT plus another investigation. Other investigations for haemorrhage, such as FAST, were performed alone on 66 patients.

With advances in CT scanning it is possible to obtain rapid and detailed information on injuries and site of haemorrhage. If CT scanning is appropriately co-located with the emergency department and suitably staffed, then this imaging modality has the potential to provide information on all but the most unstable patients. There is now emerging literature showing the use of whole body CT scanning in the multiple injured patient can reveal unsuspected injuries, locate the source of haemorrhage, speed up definitive care and reduce additional unnecessary investigations. Whole body multi-sliced CT scanning with contrast should become routine in the patient with multiple injuries. There is probably no role for chest x-ray, pelvic x-ray and other plain films if the patient is to undergo whole body CT scanning as these plain films will delay definitive investigation.

The advisors assessed the necessity of a CT scan for haemorrhage, for each patient. Table 59 shows these data and demonstrates that there was general agreement between the clinical decisions and the advisors' opinions. However, in 21/457 (4.6%) cases advisors judged that a CT scan was performed unnecessarily. In addition it was judged that in 30/309 (9.7%) cases a CT scan was indicated, but was not performed.

Table 59. Advisors' opinion on the necessity of a CT scan for haemorrhage

	CT necessary				
CT scan	**Yes**	**No**	**Subtotal**	**Insufficient data**	**Total**
Yes	436	21	**457**	26	**483**
No	30	279	**309**	3	**312**
Total	**466**	**300**	**766**	**29**	**795**

Time to CT scanning

In those cases where the time to CT scan could be determined from the casenotes, the average time taken for a CT scan after arrival in hospital was 138 minutes (2.3 hours) in those patients who only had a CT scan to investigate haemorrhage and 181 minutes (3.0 hours) in patients who had a CT scan and another investigation.

Long time delays to the CT scanner frequently occurred (Figure 27). This is likely to have major clinical implications and ultimately be detrimental to patient outcome. Therefore, hospitals admitting severely injured patients must provide more timely access to this important imaging modality.

Timeliness of CT scanning

In 55/254 cases, the clinician completing the A&E questionnaire indicated that there was a delay to CT scanning. Twenty out of these 55 delays were due the instability of the patient. The remaining 35 cases were delayed due to organisational factors.

Awaiting radiology staff was a major source of delay (Figure 28). This occurs as it is unusual for any hospital in the UK to have resident CT radiographers, unlike North America, Australasia, the Far East or mainland Europe where this would be considered normal. The lack of the timely presence of CT radiography staff is a major issue and an apparent weakness of the multidisciplinary team required to provide rapid definitive care to the severely injured patient.

Even the cases where the reason for delay was cited as 'patient instability' may be contributed to organisational factors: consultant involvement was variable (especially out of hours) and junior medical staff may have been more reticent than consultants to move potentially unstable patients to the CT scanner. Furthermore, the location of the CT scanner may

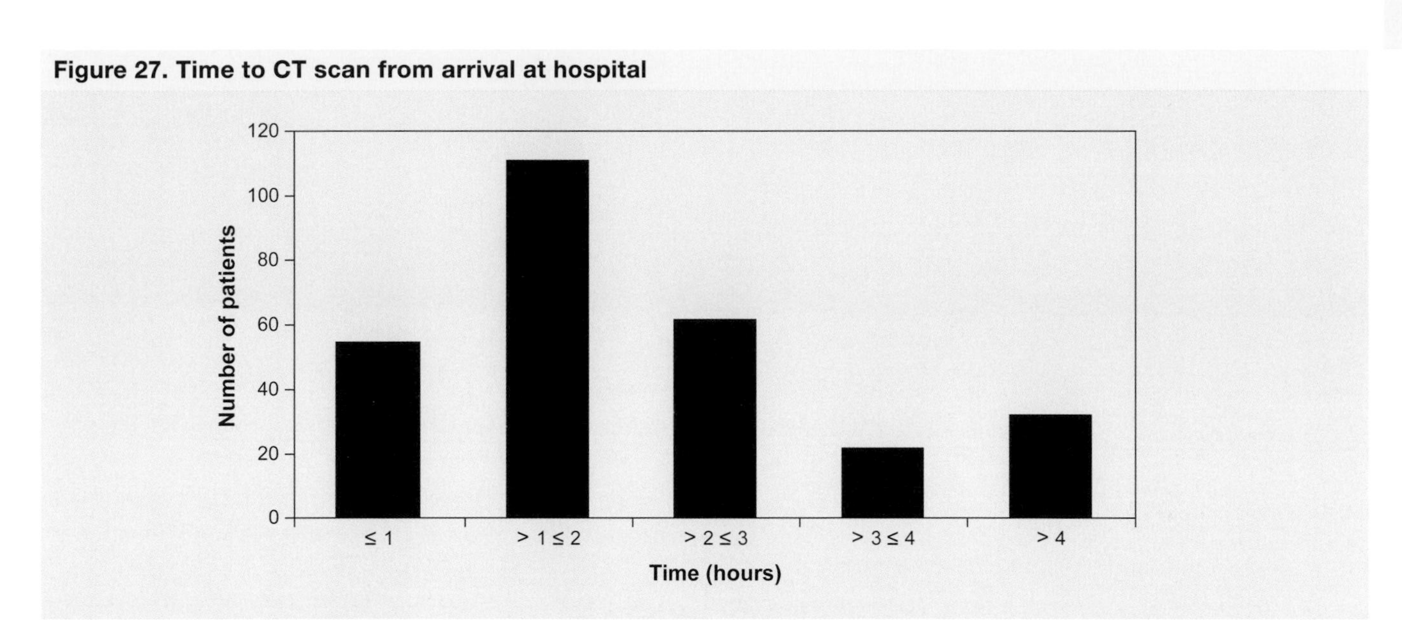

Figure 27. Time to CT scan from arrival at hospital

Figure 28. Reason for delay in CT scan (data from the A&E questionnaire)

Number of patients
25
20
15
10
5
0
Patient not stable enough
Awaiting radiology staff
Patient not stable enough and awaiting radiology staff
Awaiting access to CT
Awaiting suitable medical staff to accompany patient
Other
Not answered
Reason

change the threshold for making the clinical decision that the patient is stable enough to scan: it is clearly easier and safer if the CT scanner is close to the emergency department rather than in a remote area. In Europe, CT scanners are now being installed into resuscitation rooms within the emergency department to provide a comprehensive combined resuscitation/investigation area.

The philosophy of care that 'unstable' patients should not be taken to the CT scanner is widely accepted but not based on any evidence. It is common sense that an unstable patient (i.e. a bleeding patient) will only be stabilised by stopping the bleeding. Delaying surgery or scanning 'to wait for stabilisation' does not make sense. If the patient is considered too unstable for CT scan then transfer to theatre is required instead.

Case study 3

An elderly patient was involved in a road traffic collision. The patient arrived at hospital speaking, pulse 120 but blood pressure was unrecordable. The patient became agitated and was intubated. A chest x-ray, pelvic x-ray and abdominal ultrasound were performed. The ultrasound of the abdomen revealed a splenic injury and free fluid in the peritoneal space. The patient was then transferred to CT for chest, abdomen, head and spine. During this time the patient was unstable and received seven litres of fluid and five units of blood. Following CT scanning, the patient was transferred to critical care to be stabilised prior to laparotomy and thoracotomy. At surgery splenic and liver injuries were packed and a diaphragmatic tear repaired. The patient returned from theatre unstable despite inotropic support and subsequently arrested and died. The casenotes did not document any consultant involvement in the management of this patient and the advisors believed that this was an avoidable death.

Appropriateness of CT scanning

It was judged by the clinical advisors that a CT scan was necessary in 466 of the cases. Seventeen patients did not have a CT when the advisors thought that it was required. A further 21 cases had a CT scan but it was assessed as being unnecessary.

Reasons for assessment that the CT scan was unnecessary (21cases) were:

- **The patient was shocked with obvious intraperitoneal haemorrhage and it was felt that immediate surgery, rather than imaging, was required (five cases)**
- **FAST had revealed free fluid and it was felt that no further imaging should have been required prior to surgery (five cases)**
- **No indication for imaging (six cases)**
- **No reason was supplied for this assessment (five cases).**

Appropriateness of assessment of haemorrhage

In general it was assessed that the possibility of haemorrhage was investigated satisfactorily in 90.9% (610/671) of cases. However, in 61/671 cases (9.1%) it was considered that the possibility of haemorrhage was not investigated satisfactorily. In 124 cases there was insufficient information to assess this.

Interventions

One hundred and ten patients underwent surgery or further procedures for the control of haemorrhage.

Procedures performed to manage haemorrhage

The procedures performed to manage haemorrhage are shown in Figure 29. The majority of patients who were operated on to manage abdominal trauma – 67/110 (60.9%) required a laparotomy.

Interventional radiology has an increasing role to play in the management of the multiple trauma patient[44] and it was noted that this was undertaken in only one case.

The infrequent use of interventional radiology is likely to reflect the lack of 24 hour availability of interrentional radiology consultants who possess the necessary expertise to perform these procedures. Such factors should be considered and taken into account when planning regional trauma services.

Grade of surgeon

Fifty seven out of 73 (78%) operations, where the grade could be determined, were performed by consultants (Table 60).

Table 60. Grade of operating surgeon

	Number of patients	%
Consultant	57	78.1
SpR	16	21.9
Subtotal	**73**	
Insufficient data	37	
Total	**110**	

Figure 29. Procedure performed for haemorrhage control

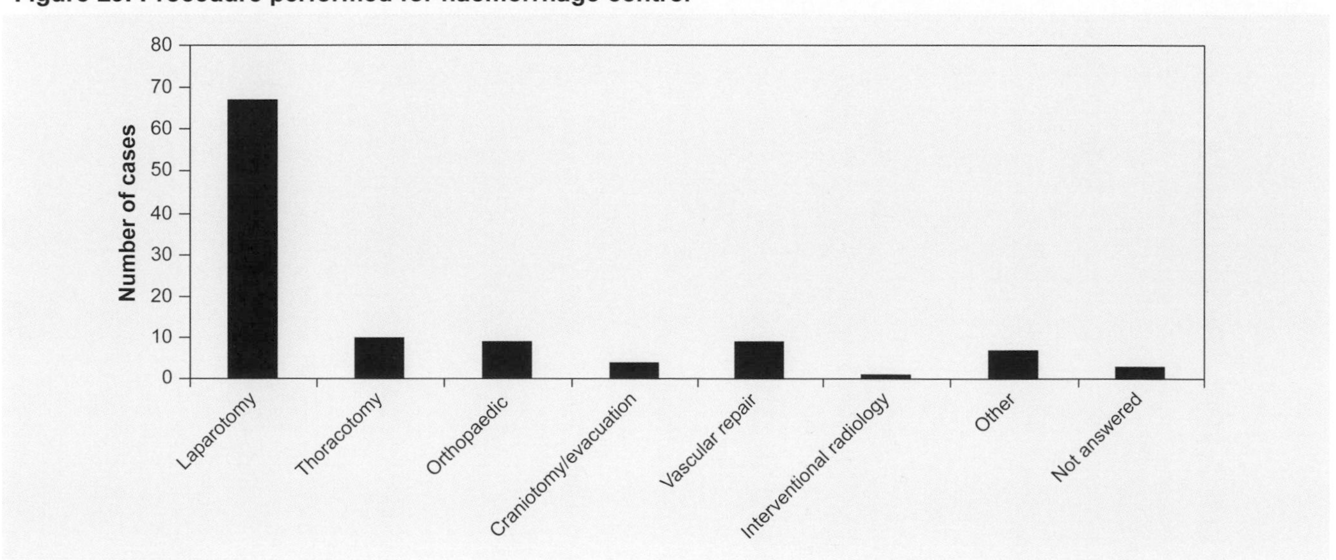

Appropriateness of surgeon

The advisors agreed that the experience of the surgeon was appropriate in 63/73 of the cases for which the grade could be determined. However, for 37/110 cases, poor documentation, particularly of the grade of the surgeon prevented judgement on the appropriateness of the surgeon's experience.

Time to surgery

It is important that definitive surgery is performed as soon as possible after admission for the trauma patient with ongoing haemorrhage.

It was possible to calculate the time to laparotomy in 51/67 cases.

The mean time to laparotomy in the whole group was 384 minutes (median 200 minutes).

The mean time to laparotomy in the group of patients who had a CT scan was 499 minutes. The mean time to laparotomy in the group of patients who did not have a CT scan was 110 minutes.

Table 61 and Figure 30 show the relationship between CT scanning and time to laparotomy.

Table 61. Time to laparotomy (hours) related to CT use

	CT scan			
	Yes	**%**	**No**	**%**
≤ 1	2	5.6	5	33.3
> 1 ≤ 2	4	11.1	6	40
> 2 ≤ 3	4	11.1	3	20
> 3 ≤ 4	8	22.2	0	
> 4	18	50	1	6.7
Total	**36**		**15**	

Figure 30. CT scan for haemorrhage and time to laparotomy

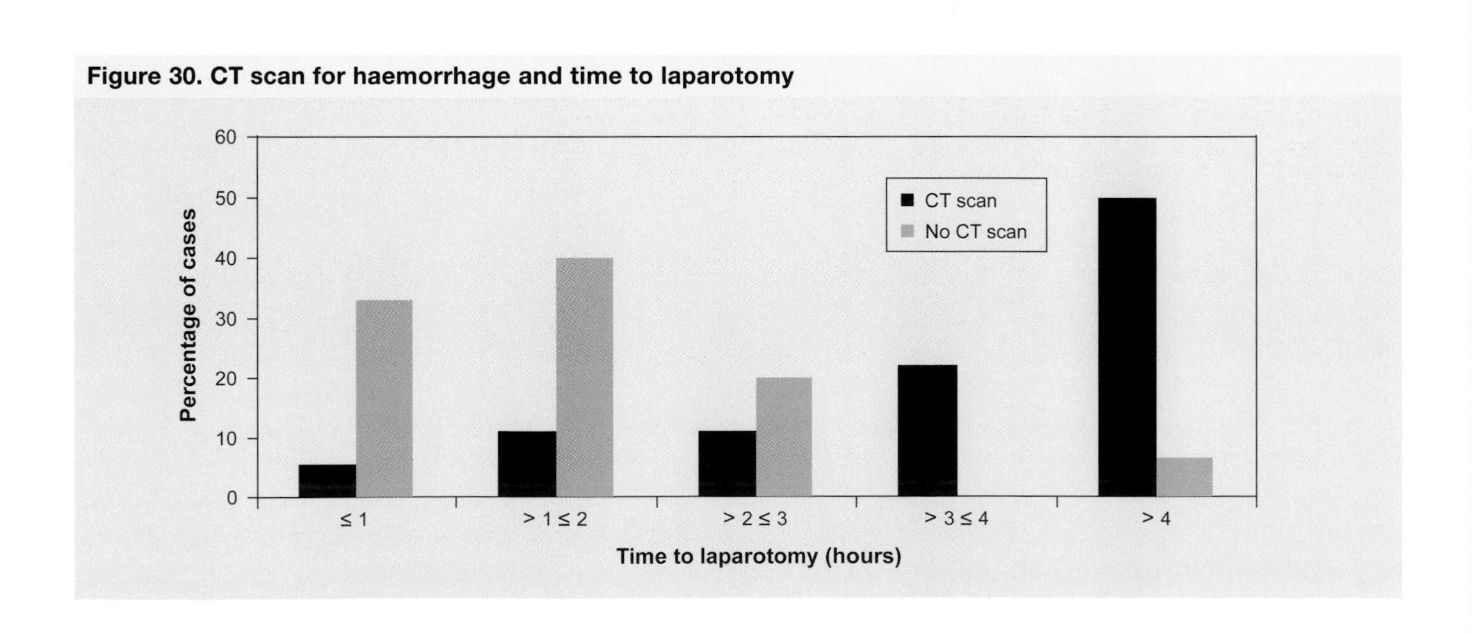

The time to trauma laparotomy in the whole group did not compare favourably to published data from a trauma centre[47]. In that study[47] median time to laparotomy was 127 minutes compared to 200 minutes in this study. It can be seen that the use of CT scanning was associated with much longer times to trauma laparotomy but the reasons behind this were not clear from the data collected.

Timeliness of surgery

The advisors were able to assess the timeliness of 87 of the 110 procedures for haemorrhage. The interventions performed were judged to be timely in 63/87 (72.4%) cases and delayed in 24/87 (27.6%) (Figure 31).

Reasons given for delays in the initiation of the procedure were multiple and often associated with the medical staff not appreciating the urgency of the requirement to control haemorrhage. Five patients were believed to have had unnecessary imaging (CT scan) as it was clear that a trauma laparotomy was required. In 12 cases it was believed that the severity of haemorrhage and urgency of the situation were not appreciated. In two cases there was a delay in provision of a staffed operating theatre.

Lack of senior involvement and lack of appreciation of clinical urgency have been found in many areas of medicine involved with acute care and the same problems have been found in trauma management.

Imaging and delays to definitive care

Table 62 shows more data for the patients who required surgery and the relationship between imaging and timeliness of operation. As can be seen from the data, it was more likely that delays were reported if imaging was performed as opposed to a clinical decision that the patient required an immediate operation. In the latter group, 19/20 patients were considered to have received timely surgery.

Figure 31. Procedure performed was timely (advisors' view)

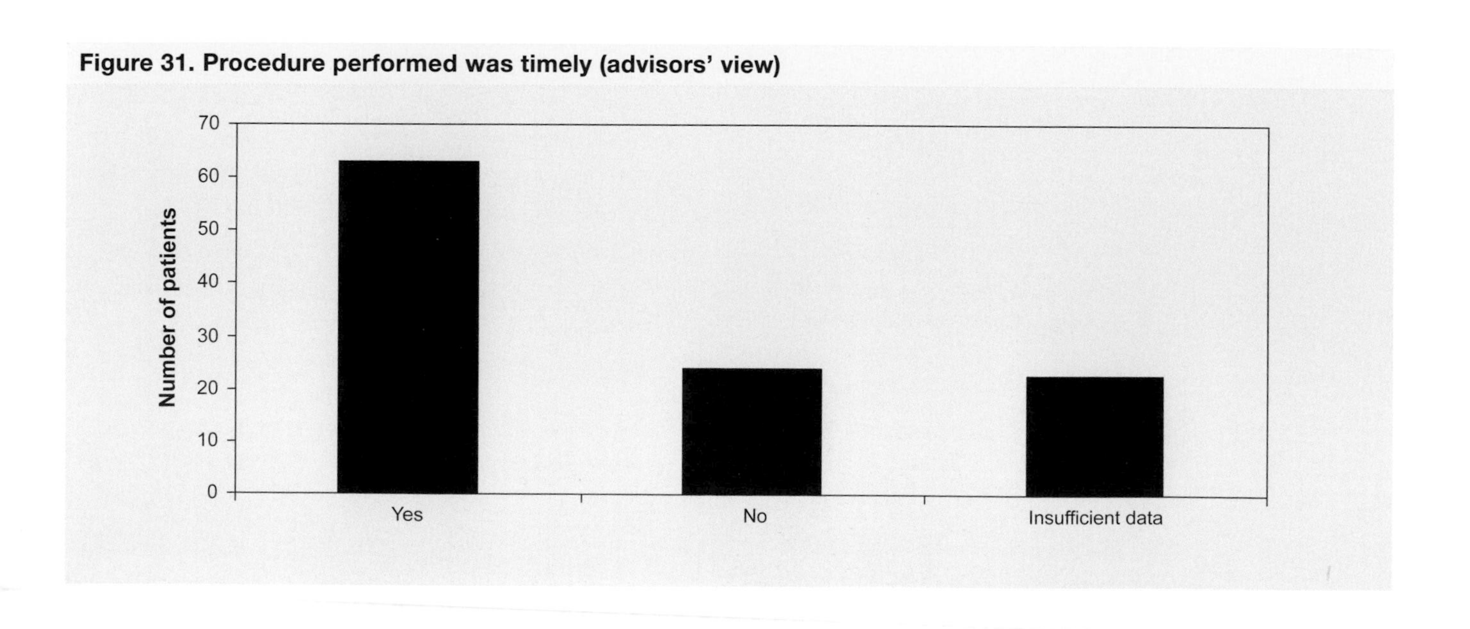

Table 62. Timely procedure for imaging for haemorrhage

	Imaging for haemorrhage				
Procedure timely	**CT**	**CT & Other**	**Other**	**None**	**Total**
Yes	24	9	11	19	**63**
No	12	5	6	1	**24**
Subtotal	**36**	**14**	**17**	**20**	**87**
Insufficient data	15	3	2	3	**23**
Total	**51**	**17**	**19**	**23**	**110**

Imaging has a major role to play in the management of the severely injured patient. However, as assessment must be rapid and accurate, imaging should be appropriate and the choice of modality should reflect which is more likely to give a rapid diagnosis. Inappropriate application of imaging or delays in accessing imaging may delay definitive care.

Operative management – summary

It is clear from the above that there are concerns about the operative management of the trauma patient. Whilst 78.1% of patients for whom the grade of surgeon could be determined were operated on by a consultant, in 37 cases requiring an intervention for haemorrhage there was no documentation of the surgeon's grade. In 27.6% of cases it was felt that the operation was not performed in a timely fashion.

Outcome for patients requiring surgery

In this sample 72 hour mortality for patients who had surgery was 22.7% (25/110) whereas for those who did not have surgery for haemorrhage it was 13.7% (92/670).

It was observed that for those patients who had timely intervention to control bleeding the 72 hour mortality was 23.8% (15/63) compared with 33.3% (8/24) where the intervention was considered delayed.

Overall management

The overall management of the patients' haemorrhage was considered satisfactory by the advisors in 412/462 (89.2%). More importantly, 50/462 (10.8%) cases were identified as not having satisfactory management of haemorrhage. No assessment was made by the advisors on the remaining 333 cases, presumably as there was no clinical indication for haemorrhage in these patients.

Overall management – operated cases

Table 63 shows that 19/98 patients who required an operation were considered to have unsatisfactory management.

Table 63. Overall management of haemorrhage was satisfactory

	Number of patients	%
Yes	79	80.6
No	19	19.4
Subtotal	**98**	
Insufficient data	12	
Total	**110**	

In summary, there appeared to be problems with the investigation and control of haemorrhage. The areas of concern were principally the rapid recognition of haemorrhage and the institution of definitive management. There appeared to be delays to laparotomy and lack of initial consultant input.

The inability to rapidly CT scan trauma patients may relate to the proximity of the CT scanner to the emergency department. Locating the scanner adjacent to, or as part of, the resuscitation suite may rectify this problem. We also note the limited use of interventional radiology in the management of bleeding patients. There is evidence that increased use of interventional radiology plays an important role in the management of blood loss in the severely injured patient and that integration of radiology staff and resources into the trauma system may improve patient outcomes[44].

Key findings

51.3% (254/495) of the patients had a CT scan of the chest, abdomen and pelvis for assessment of blood loss.

In 55/254 (21.7%) cases there was a delay to CT scanning.

In 61/671 cases (9.1%) it was felt that the possibility of haemorrhage was not investigated satisfactorily.

110/795 patients (13.8%) underwent surgery or further procedures for the control of haemorrhage.

57/73 (78.1%) operations were performed by consultants.

In 37/110 (33.6%) poor documentation prevented the grade of the surgeon being determined.

The interventions performed were considered untimely in 27.6% (24/87) of patients.

Where operative intervention for haemorrhage was considered timely the 72 hour mortality was 23.8% (15/63) compared to 33.3% (8/24) where the intervention was considered delayed.

19/98 (19.4%) patients from whom data were available and who required surgery for management of haemorrhage had unsatisfactory overall management.

Recommendations

Rapid identification of patients who require immediate surgery for control of haemorrhage is essential. Ongoing fluid requirements and instability identify a group of patients who require immediate intervention rather than further investigation. Local protocols should clearly identify the patient population for whom it is inappropriate to delay the surgery/intervention for reasons of 'stabilisation' or further investigation. *(Hospital trusts, clinical directors and emergency physicians)*

Trauma laparotomy is potentially extremely challenging and requires consultant presence within the operating theatre. *(Clinical directors)*

CT scanning will have an increasing role in the investigation and management of trauma patients. In major centres, CT facilities should be co-located with the emergency department to provide a combined investigation/resuscitation area. *(Hospital trusts)*

If CT scanning is to be performed, all necessary images should be obtained at the same time. Routine use of 'top to toe' scanning is recommended in the adult trauma patient if no indication for immediate intervention exists. *(Royal College of Radiology and radiology department heads)*

Timely access to CT scanning is essential. CT radiographers should be available within 30 minutes of the patient arriving in hospital. In larger trauma centres, with a higher workload, CT radiographers should be immediately available at all times.

In the setting of remote radiology facilities and/or lack of timely access to CT scanning, unstable patients should not be taken to the CT scanner. These unstable patients should have immediate surgery. *(Trauma team leader)*

References

1. Shackford SR, Mackersie RC, Holbrook TL, et al. *The epidemiology of traumatic death: A population-based analysis.* Arch Surg 1993;128:571
2. Sauaia A, Moore FA, Moore EE, et al. *Epidemiology of trauma deaths: A reassessment.* J Trauma 1995;38:185-193
3. Champion HR, Copes WS, Sacco WJ, Lawnick MM, Keast SL, Bain LW, Flanagan ME, Frey CF. *The Major Trauma Outcome Study: Establishing National Norms for Trauma Care.* J Trauma 1990; 30: 1356-1365
4. Marmarou A, Anderson RL, Ward JD, et al. *Impact on ICP instability and hypotension on outcome in patients with severe head trauma.* J Neurosurg 1991;75(suppl):S59-S66
5. Chestnut RM, Marshall LF, Klauber MR, et al. *The role of secondary brain injury in determining outcome from severe head injury.* J Trauma 1993;34:216-222
6. Goins WA, Reynolds HN, Nyanjom D, et al. *Outcome following prolonged intensive care unit stay in multiple trauma patients.* Crit Care Med 1991;19:339
7. Moore FA, Moore EE. *Evolving concepts in the pathogenesis of postinjury multiple organ failure.* Surg Clin North Am 1995;75:257
8. Jurkovich GJ, Greiser WB, Lyterman A, et al. *Hypothermia in trauma victims: an ominous predictor of survival.* J Trauma 1987;27:1019-1024
9. Luna GK, Maier RV, Pavlin EG, et al. *Incidence and effect of hypothermia in seriously injured patients.* J Trauma 1987;27:1014-1017

10. Reed RL, Bracey AW, Hudson JD, et al. *Hypothermia and blood coagulation: dissociation between enzyme activity and clotting factor levels.* Circ Shock 1990;32:141-152

11. Schreiber MA. *Damage control surgery.* Crit Care Clin 2004;20:101-118

12. MacLeod JB, Lynn M, McKenny MG, et al. *Early coagulopathy predicts mortality in trauma.* J Trauma 2003;55:39-44

13. Cosgriff N, Moore EE, Sauaia A, et al. *Predicting life-threatening coagulopathy in the massively transfused patient: hypothermia and acidosis revisited.* J Trauma 1997;42:857-62

14. Hill DA, West RH, Roncal S. *Outcome of patients with haemorrhagic shock: an indicator of performance in a trauma centre.* J R Coll Surg Edinb 1995;40:221-4

15. Spahn DR, Cerny V, Coats TJ, et al. *Management of bleeding patients following major trauma: A European guideline.* Criti Care 2007;11:R17

16. Demetriades D, Chan L, Cornwell E, et al. *Paramedic vs. private transportation of trauma patients. Effect on outcome.* Arch Surg. 1996;131:133-8

17. Gervin AS, Fischer RP. *The importance of prompt transport of salvage patients with penetrating heart wounds.* J Trauma 1982;22:443-8

18. Gold CR. *Prehospital advanced life support vs. 'scoop and run' in trauma management.* Ann Emerg Med. 1987;16:797-801

19. Feero S, Hedges JR, Simmons E, Irwin L. *Does out-of-hospital EMS time affect survival?* Am J Emerg Med. 1995;13:133-5

20. Regel G, Stalp M, Lehmann U, Seekamp A. *Prehospital care, importance of early intervention on outcome.* Acta Anaesthesiol Scand. 1997;110(Suppl.):71-6

21. Ruteledge R, Fakhry SM, Meyer A, Sheldon GF, Baker CC. *An analysis of the association of trauma centres with per capita hospitalisations and death rates from injury.* Ann Surg 1993;218:512-24

22. Eastman AB, Schwab CW, Annest JL, et al. *Position paper on trauma care systems.* J Trauma 1992;32:127-9

23. Shackford SR, Mackersie RC, Hoyt DB, et al. *Impact of a trauma system on outcome of severely injured patients.* Arch Surg 1987; 122:523-7

24. MacKenzie EJ, Rivara FP, Jurkovich GJ, et al. *A national evaluation of the effect of trauma-center care on mortality.* N Engl J Med. 2006;354:366-78

25. West JG, Trunkey DD, Lim RC. *Systems of trauma care: A study of two counties.* Arch Surg 1979;114:455

26. Lowe DK, Gately HL, Goss JR, et al. *Patterns of death, complication and error in the management of motor accident victims: Implications for a regional system of trauma care.* J Trauma 1983;23:503

27. Van Wagoner FH. *A three year study of deaths following trauma.* J Trauma 1961;1:401

28. Tien HC, Spencer F, Tremblay LN, Rizoli SB, Brenneman FD. *Preventable deaths from hemorrhage at a level 1 Canadian trauma center.* J Trauma. 2007; 62: 142-6

29. Porter JM, Ivatury RR. *In search of the optimal end points of resuscitation in trauma: a review.* J Trauma 1998;44:908-14

30. Revell M, Greaves I, Porter K. *Endpoints for fluid resuscitation in hemorrhagic shock.* J Trauma 2003;54:S63-S67

31. Vincent JL, Dufaye P, Berre J, et al. *Serial lactate determinations during circulatory shock.* Crit Care Med 1983;11:449-451

32. Abramson D, Scalea TM, Hitchcock R, et al. *Lactate clearance and survival following injury.* J Trauma 1993;35:584-589

33. Davis JW, Kaups KL, Parks SN. *Base deficit is superior to pH in evaluating clearance of acidosis after traumatic shock.* J Trauma 1998;44:114-118

34. Davis JW, Shackford SR, MacKersie RC, Hoyt DB. *Base deficit as a guide to volume resuscitation.* J Trauma 1988;28:1464-1467

35. Davis JW, Kaups KL. *Base deficit in the elderly: a marker of severe injury and death.* J Trauma 1998;45:873-877

36. Fitzsullivan E, Salim A, Demetriades D, et al. *Serum bicarbonate may replace the arterial base deficit in the trauma intensive care unit.* Am J Surg 2005;190:961-967

37. Porter RS, Nester BA, Dalsey WC. *Use of ultrasound to determine need for laparotomy in trauma patients.* Ann Emerg Med 1997;29:323-330

38. Rozycki GS, Ochsner MG, Schmidt JA, et al. *A prospective study of surgeon-performed ultrasound as the primary adjuvant modality for injured patient assessment.* J Trauma 1995;39:492-498

39. Stengel D, Bauwens K, Sehouli J, et al. *Systematic review and meta-analysis of emergency ultrasounography for blunt abdominal trauma.* Br J Surg 2001;88:901-912

40. Velmahos GC, Toutouzas KG, Radin R, Chan L, Demetriades D. *Nonoperative treatment of blunt injury to solid organs. A prospective study.* Arch Surg 2003;138:844-851

41. Velmahos GC, Toutouzas KG, Radin R, Chan L, Rhee P, Tillou A, Demetriades D. *High success with nonoperative management of blunt hepatic trauma. The liver is a sturdy organ.* Arch Surg 2003;138:475-481

42. Cook RE, Keating JF, Gillespie I: *The role of angiography in the management of haemorrhage from major fractures of the pelvis.* J Bone Joint Surg Br 2002;84:178-182

43. Hamill J, Holden A, Paice R, et al. *Pelvic fracture pattern predicts pelvic arterial haemorrhage.* Aust N Z J Surg 2000;70:338-343

44. Pryor JP, Braslow B, Reilly PM, Gullamondegi O, Hendrick JH, Schwab CW. *The evolving role of interventional radiology in trauma care.* J Trauma 2005;59:102-4

45. Rotondo M, Schwab CW, McGonigal M, et al. *Damage control: an approach for improved survival in exsanguinating penetrating abdominal injury.* J Trauma 1993;35:375-383

46. Shapiro MB, Jenkins DH, Schwab CW, et al. *Damage Control: collective review.* J Trauma 2000;49:969-978

47. Henderson KI, Coats TJ, Hassan TB, Brohi K. *Audit of time to trauma laparotomy.* Br J Surg 2000; 87:472-476

CHAPTER 8 - Head injury management

Introduction

In the UK, traumatic brain injury accounts for 15-20% of deaths between the ages of 5 and 35 years, with an incidence of 9 per 100 000 per year[1]. Outcome after head injury depends upon the initial severity of injury and also the extent of any subsequent complications and how these are managed. Most of the patients who attend hospital after a head injury do not develop life threatening or disabling complications in the acute stage. However, in a small but important group of patients, outcome is made worse by a failure to detect promptly or to deal adequately with complications[2-7].

There is a growing body of evidence that secondary insults occur frequently and exert a profound, adverse effect on outcome from severe head injury. It is therefore recommended that hypotension (Systolic BP <90mmHg) and hypoxia (PaO_2 <8kPa) must be scrupulously avoided or treated immediately to avoid worsening outcome[8].

The use of guidelines in the early management of head injuries was endorsed by a Department of Health seminar in 1983 and has been supported many times over the last two decades[9-15]. More recently, comprehensive guidelines have been produced by the Scottish Intercollegiate Guidelines Network (SIGN Guideline 46)[16] and the National Institute for Health and Clinical Excellence (NICE)[17]. There is, therefore, no shortage of guidelines for the management of patients who have suffered a head injury and it should be expected that current practice would be informed by this literature.

Results

Incidence of neurotrauma

Of the 795 patients within the study, 493 (62.0%) had suffered neurotrauma as part of their constellation of injuries.

Impact of neurotrauma

Table 64 shows the patient location at 72 hours after admission to hospital. In this sample more patients with neurotrauma were deceased at 72 hours when compared to the rest of the sample.

Table 64. Patient location at 72 hours

	Head injury		Non head injury		Whole sample	
		%		%		%
Level 3 care	158	35.7	81	30.9	239	33.9
Specialist ward	83	18.8	59	22.5	142	20.2
Deceased	87	19.7	30	11.5	117	16.6
Level 2 care	29	6.6	35	13.4	64	9.1
General ward	25	5.7	35	13.4	60	8.5
Transferred, outcome unknown	39	8.8	17	6.5	56	8.0
Home	18	4.1	3	1.1	21	3.0
Other	3	<1	2	<1	5	<1
Subtotal	**442**		**262**		**704**	
Not documented	51		40		91	
Total	**493**		**302**		**795**	

In addition to a higher 72 hour mortality, head injured patients required more critical care resources than non-head injured patients.

Prehospital data

Assessment of neurological function

Figure 32 and Table 65 show the prehospital assessment of conscious level in the patients who had suffered a head injury. It should be noted that a patient report form (PRF) was available for 320 of the 493 head injury group.

Most patients had a Glasgow Coma Score (GCS) calculated, although some prehospital assessment was performed using the AVPU (Alert, Verbal, Pain, Unresponsive) scale. Eighteen patients had no assessment of neurological dysfunction.

Table 65. AVPU score in head injury group

	Number of patients	%
Alert	27	34.6
Verbal	18	23.1
Pain	13	16.7
Unresponsive	20	25.6
Subtotal	**78**	
GCS and/or AVPU not recorded	18	
Total	**96**	

It is important to document neurological status so that any changes can be recognised and acted upon. Pupil size and reactivity should also be recorded when assessment of conscious level is being made. NICE guidance recommends that the GCS should be used in all communications about head injured patients and that ambulance crews should be fully trained in the adult and paediatric versions of the Glasgow Coma Scale[17].

Figure 32. Prehospital Glasgow Coma Score measurement in head injury group

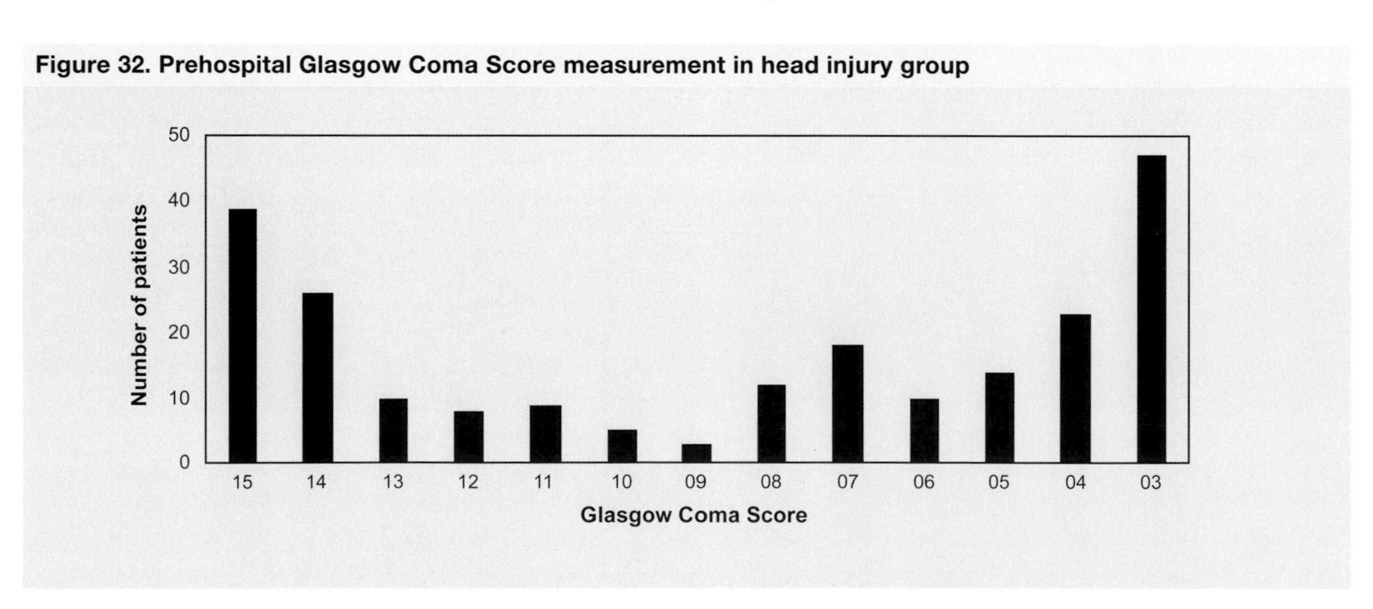

Table 66. Prehospital SpO_2 (%) measurements

	Alive	Deceased	Total	% Mortality
Unrecordable	1	4	5	80
< 80	6	4	10	40
≥ 80 < 85	9	5	14	35.7
≥ 85 < 90	9	4	13	30.7
≥ 90 < 95	24	5	29	17.2
≥ 95 < 100	95	19	114	16.7
100	47	8	55	14.5
Subtotal	**191**	**49**	**240**	**20.4**
Not recorded	65	15	80	18.8
Total	**256**	**64**	**320**	**20**

Oxygen therapy and oxygenation

Oxygen therapy is considered basic care in the severely injured patient. This is particularly relevant to the head injured patient where hypoxia significantly increases the risk of mortality[18-20].

Oxygen therapy was administered to only 78.1% (250/320) of patients with neurotrauma.

Table 66 shows the prehospital SpO_2 measurements. There were substantial numbers of patients who were profoundly hypoxaemic in the prehospital phase. In this study 37/240 (15.4%) patients had SpO_2 <90% and 66/240 (27.5%) patients had SpO_2 <95% which is known to have a significant negative impact on patient outcome.

Given the high incidence of hypoxia it was of particular note that almost a quarter of patients, for whom data were available, did not receive oxygen prior to arrival at hospital.

Airway management

Intubation and ventilatory support is often required to reverse hypoxia and hypoventilation. Table 67 shows that 48 patients were intubated in the prehospital setting and that seven had attempted but failed intubation.

Table 67. Prehospital intubation

	Number of patients	%
Yes	48	15.0
No	265	82.8
Failed attempt	7	2.2
Subtotal	**320**	
Patient Report Form not included	173	
Total	**493**	

Of the 265 patients not intubated in the prehospital phase, 162 were intubated in hospital. A total of 72/162 (44.4%) were intubated either on admission to hospital or within the first 30 minutes.

The patients who required prehospital intubation might well have been more severely injured (hence the need for advanced airway intervention). Table 68 shows outcome data at 72 hours post injury in the head injured patients.

Table 68. Outcome at 72 hours by intubation in the prehospital phase

	Not intubated		Intubated		Failed attempt	
		%		%		%
Alive	225	84.9	30	62.5	1	14.3
Deceased	40	15.1	18	37.5	6	85.7
Total	**265**		**48**		**7**	

The intubated group had a higher mortality than the non-intubated group (37.5% v 15.1%). The failed intubation group had a mortality rate of 85.7%. Although these are very small numbers this group had a much worse outcome.

Airway intervention and Glasgow Coma Score

Figure 33 and table 69 relate airway intervention to prehospital assessment of conscious level. The greater the degree of neurological injury, the greater the likelihood of the need for intubation. All but two of the patients who had a failed intubation attempt had a GCS of 3.

Table 69. AVPU score by intubation

	Not intubated	Intubated	Failed attempt
Alert	0	0	0
Verbal	0	0	0
Pain	8	4	1
Unresponsive	13	7	0
Total	**21**	**11**	**1**

Tables 70 and 71 show advisors' assessment of prehospital airway and ventilation management. In the opinion of the advisors, all measures were taken to secure an adequate airway in 234/273 cases and all measures to ensure

Figure 33. Prehospital Glasgow Coma Score and intubation for the head injury group

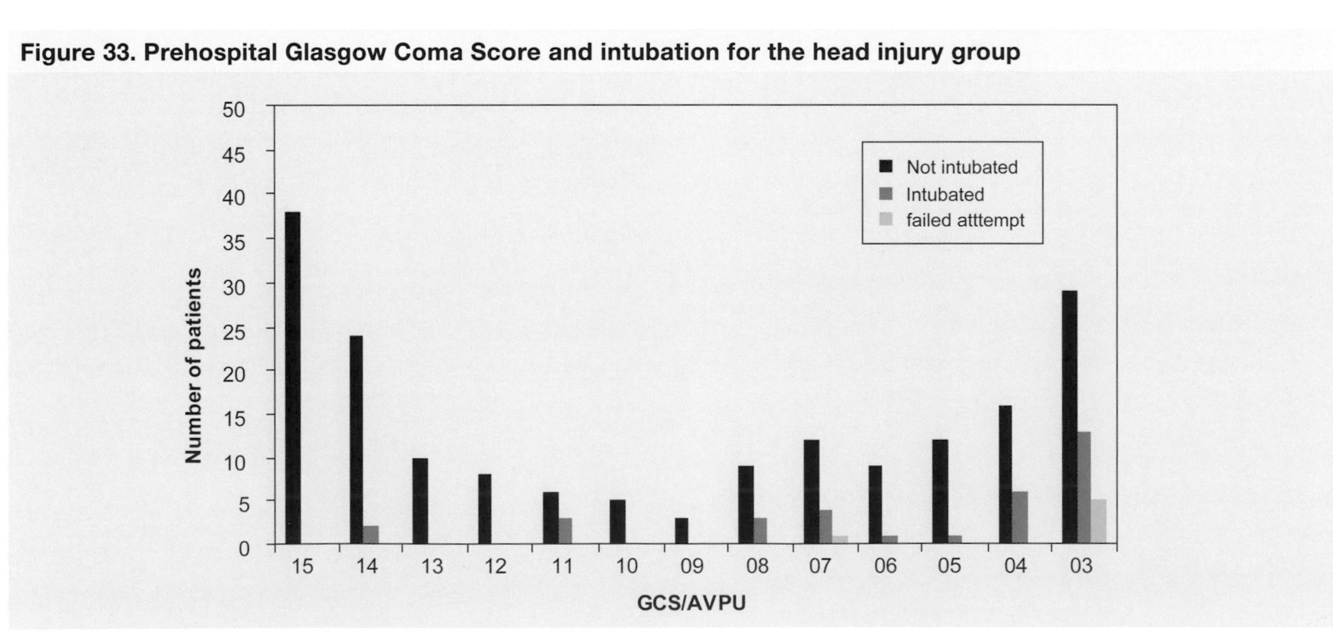

adequate ventilation in 245/274 cases where sufficient data were available to make these assessments. This means that there were concerns with airway management in 39 (14.3%) cases and ventilatory management in 29 (10.6%) cases.

Table 70. Adequate airway

	Number of patients	%
Yes	234	85.7
No	39	14.3
Subtotal	**273**	
Insufficient data	47	
Total	**320**	

Table 71. Adequate ventilation

	Number of patients	%
Yes	245	89.4
No	29	10.6
Subtotal	**274**	
Insufficient data	46	
Total	**320**	

This incidence of inadequate airway management does not fit with the current guidelines for the management of severe head injury which state that patients who have suffered severe head injury should be intubated and receive ventilatory support. From Figure 33, 103 patients with GCS less than 9 were not intubated prior to arrival at hospital. It may be that the advisors did not include all the unintubated patients in the inadequate airway management group as they were aware of the constraints of the current prehospital paramedic based system (with respect to ability to anaesthetise and intubate patients).

Despite the above comments on the advisors' opinion of the incidence of airway problems, and the possible under reporting of this issue, Table 72 shows that the 72 hour mortality rate more than doubled for the group of patients that advisors judged had received inadequate airway or ventilatory management prehospital.

These data serve to underline the importance of adequate airway control and avoidance of hypoxia and hypercapnia.

Table 72. Adequate airway/ventilation by outcome at 72 hours

	Adequate airway				Adequate ventilation			
	Yes	**%**	**No**	**%**	**Yes**	**%**	**No**	**%**
Alive	192	82.1	23	59.0	199	81.2	16	55.2
Deceased	42	17.9	16	41.0	46	18.8	13	44.8
Total	**234**		**39**		**245**		**29**	

There is a consistent message throughout this report that significant problems are encountered in prehospital airway management:

- **Many patients arrived at hospital with an obstructed or partially obstructed airway,**
- **There was a high rate of failed intubation in the prehospital phase,**
- **Most patients with acute severe head injury were transported to hospital unintubated,**
- **There was a high incidence of hypoxia and hypercapnia on admission to hospital,**
- **Many patients were intubated in the immediate period after admission to hospital.**

It is known from the literature and has been shown in this study that these problems are associated with a higher mortality rate. This implies that there is the need to routinely make available individuals with the skills and ability to provide anaesthesia and intubation to severely injured patients in the prehospital phase. This is likely to require the inclusion of physicians in the prehospital response team.

Blood pressure and cerebral perfusion

While the desirable level of blood pressure in the bleeding multiple trauma patient is subject to some debate, it is clear that hypotension worsens neurological outcome. Cerebral perfusion in patients with traumatic brain injury is critically dependent on systemic blood pressure. The minimum acceptable level of systolic blood pressure recommended by the Brain Trauma Foundation[20] is 90mmHg but even this is insufficient to maintain an adequate cerebral perfusion pressure in the case of cerebral injury. The existence of both hypoxia and hypotension in patients with traumatic brain injury is associated with a mortality rate of 75%[20].

Table 73 shows the prehospital systolic blood pressure in the head injured patients. In 21/241 (8.7%) patients a systolic blood pressure less than the minimum level suggested by the Brain Trauma Foundation was recorded.

Table 73. Systolic blood pressure (mmHg)

	Number of patients	%
< 90	21	8.7
> 90 ≤ 120	72	29.9
>120	148	61.4
Subtotal	**241**	
Not Recorded	79	
Total	**320**	

Hospital data

Pre-alerts

Pre-alerts allow the emergency department to provide a rapid and appropriate response. In the head injured patient, where there is very strong linkage between avoidance of secondary injury and good outcome, this rapid and appropriate response is particularly important. Figure 34 shows the use of pre-alerts analysed by prehospital GCS.

The use of pre-alerts was variable. Even in the patient group with a GCS of 8 or less (severe head injury) there were a substantial number of patients arriving at hospital without a pre-alert. Indeed, in the group with a GCS of 3, 22.4% (17/76) of patients arrived at hospital without a pre-alert.

NICE guidance on this aspect of care states[17]:

"Standby calls to the destination A&E Department should be made for all patients with a GCS less than or equal to 8, to ensure appropriately experienced professionals are available for their treatment and to prepare for imaging".

Data from this study showed that practice was falling well short of this guideline. Fifty nine out of 160 (36.9%) patients, in which it was recorded, with severe head injury did not have a pre-alert. Delays to the amelioration of secondary insults, imaging and definitive surgery (if required) could adversely affect outcome.

Figure 34. Prehospital Glasgow Coma Score and documentation of an ambulance pre-alert

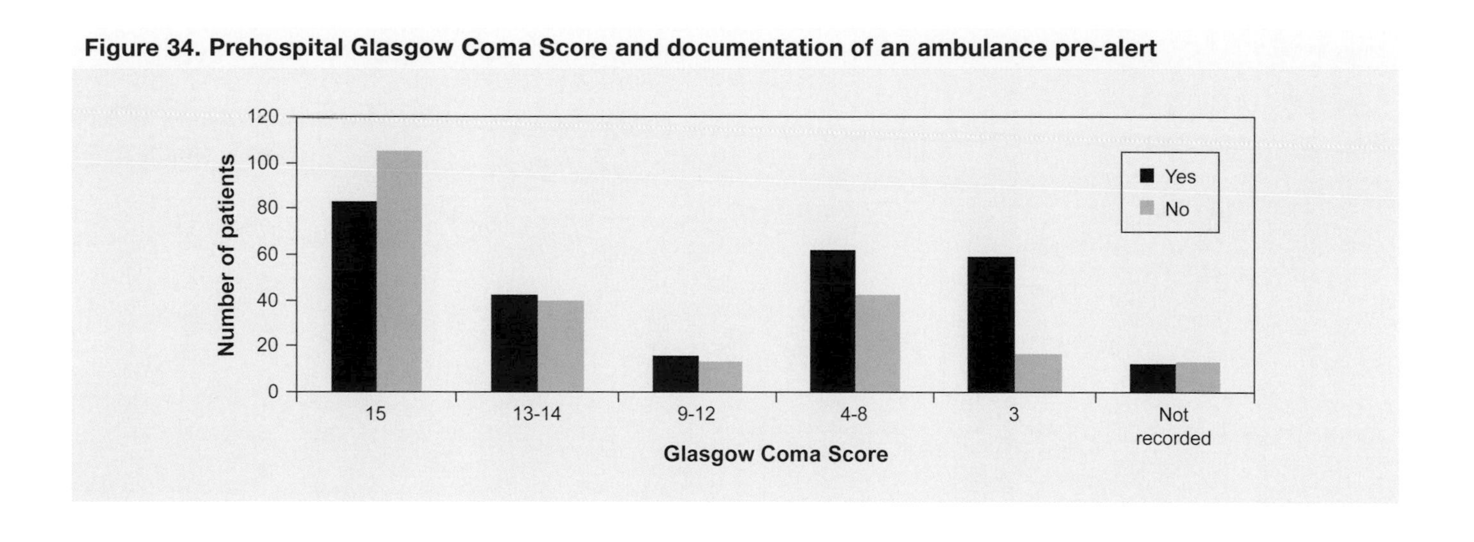

Assessment of neurological function on admission

Figure 35 shows the first documented hospital GCS in the group of patients who had suffered a head injury.

From Figure 35 it can be seen that 91 patients had minor head injury (GCS 15), 99 had mild head injury (GCS 13-14), 63 had moderate head injury (GCS 9-12) and 215 had severe head injury (GCS 3-8). Of these, 100 were first assessed to be completely unresponsive (GCS 3). For the remaining 25 patients a GCS was not documented.

The 72 hour mortality rate for each group is shown in Table 74. The group of patients with GCS 3 had a much worse outcome. It is well known that initial GCS is an independent predictor of outcome.

Table 74. Mortality rate by Glasgow Coma Score

Glasgow Coma Score	Alive	Deceased	Total	% Mortality
03	51	49	**100**	49.0
04-08	98	17	**115**	14.8
09-12	56	7	**63**	11.1
13-14	97	2	**99**	2.0
15	87	4	**91**	4.4
Subtotal	**389**	**79**	**468**	**16.9**
Not recorded	17	8	**25**	32.0
Total	**406**	**87**	**493**	**17.6**

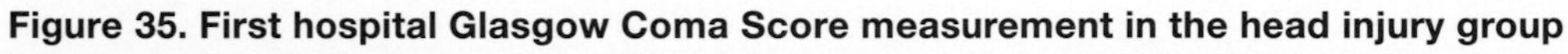

Figure 35. First hospital Glasgow Coma Score measurement in the head injury group

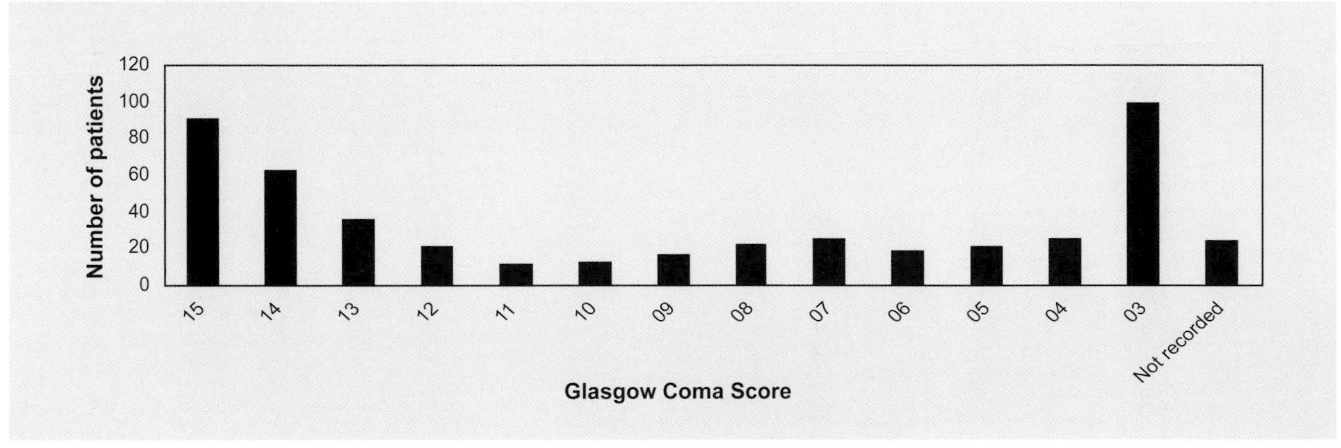

Frequency of neurological assessment

NICE guidance on this aspect of head injury management states[17]:

> "For patients admitted for head injury observation the minimum acceptable documented neurological observations are: GCS; pupil size and reactivity; limb movements; respiratory rate; heart rate; blood pressure; temperature; blood oxygen saturation. Observations should be performed and recorded on a half-hourly basis until GCS equal to 15 has been achieved."

Frequent assessment of neurological function is a key part of the management of the head injured patient. Rapid detection of deterioration is important to allow timely investigation and intervention, if required. Table 75 shows how often a GCS was documented in the first four hours after admission to hospital.

Table 75. Frequency of Glasgow Coma Score measurements during the first four hours after admission

	Number of patients	%
0	41	8.3
1	92	18.7
2	98	19.9
3	73	14.8
4	44	8.9
5	29	5.9
6	27	5.5
7	18	3.7
8	13	2.6
> 8	58	11.8
Total	**493**	

While data was not collected about time to normalisation of GCS in this study, it appears from Table 75 that the frequency of observations may have been falling far short of this NICE recommendation, as there is the opportunity to perform eight sets of observations in the first four hours.

Airway status on admission

Table 76 shows airway status on admission to hospital for the head injured group. Sixty six patients arrived at hospital with either a partially or completely obstructed airway. This represented 18.3% of the non-intubated patients (66/361).

Table 76. Airway status on arrival for the head injury group

	Number of patients	%
Clear	295	69.7
Noisy	31	7.3
Blocked	35	8.3
Intubated	62	14.7
Subtotal	**423**	
Not recorded	70	
Total	**493**	

Airway management in hospital

Many of these problems were addressed after arrival to hospital but there were 37 patients for whom the advisors felt that management of the airway and/or ventilation was unsatisfactory in hospital (Table 77). These were primarily concerns over lack of timely intubation and control of ventilation.

Table 77. Overall airway management satisfactory

	Number of patients	%
Yes	417	91.9
No	37	8.1
Subtotal	**454**	
Insufficient data	39	
Total	**493**	

After admission, mortality at 72 hours in the groups with satisfactory and unsatisfactory airway management was 73/417 (17.5%) and 10/37 (27.0%) respectively.

There were a substantial number of patients who had less than satisfactory management of airway and ventilation in both the prehospital and hospital phase. These findings indicate the potential for secondary insults to occur. The mortality rate in the unsatisfactory group supported this.

Admission pulse oximetry and blood gas analysis

Table 78 shows data on first SpO_2 measurements in hospital. Slightly more than one in ten patients were hypoxaemic (SpO_2 <95%) despite prehospital treatment.

Table 78. SpO_2 (%) measurements in hospital

	Number of patients	%
< 80	8	1.8
≥ 80 < 85	10	2.3
≥ 85 < 90	7	1.6
≥ 90 < 95	32	7.4
≥ 95 < 100	184	42.4
100	193	44.5
Subtotal	**434**	
Not recorded	59	
Total	**493**	

Figures 36, 37 and 38 show the results of the first arterial blood gas (ABG) analysis after hospital admission. As can be seen there were small, but appreciable, numbers of patients who have significant hypoxia (PaO_2 <10kPa), hypercapnia ($PaCO_2$ >6kPa), hypocapnia ($PaCO_2$ <4kPa) and acidosis (pH <7.35). There were also a large number of cases where no ABG analysis was performed (202/493).

Figure 36. First documented ABG PaO_2 measurement

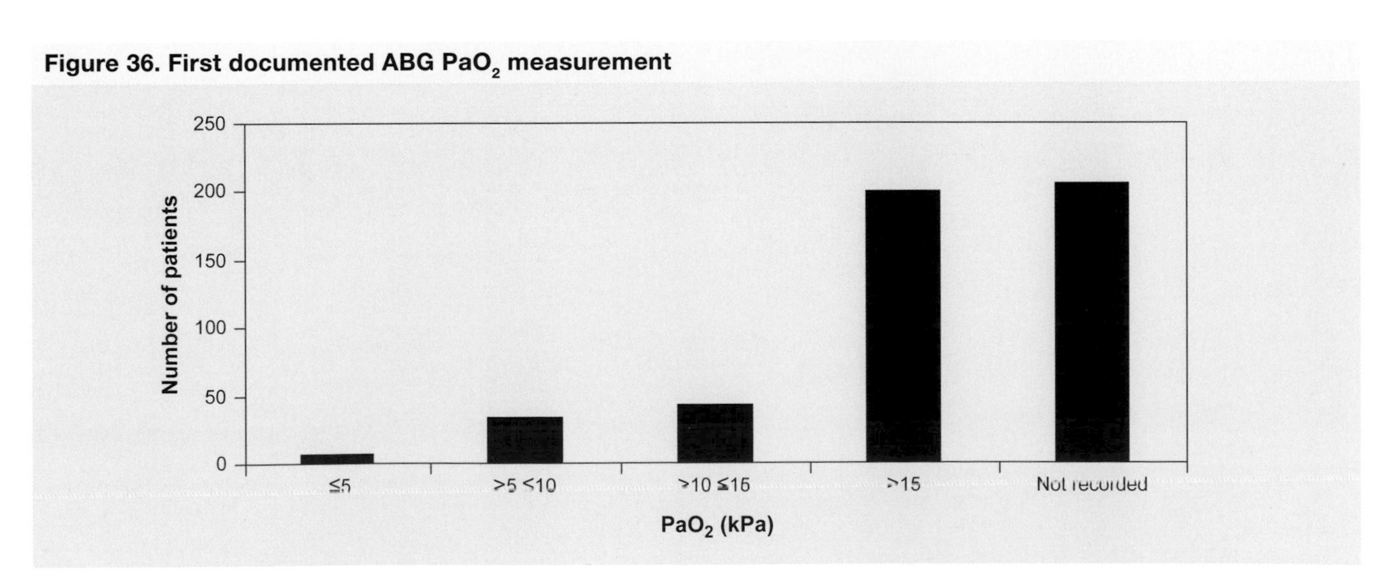

Figure 37. First documented ABG $PaCO_2$ measurement

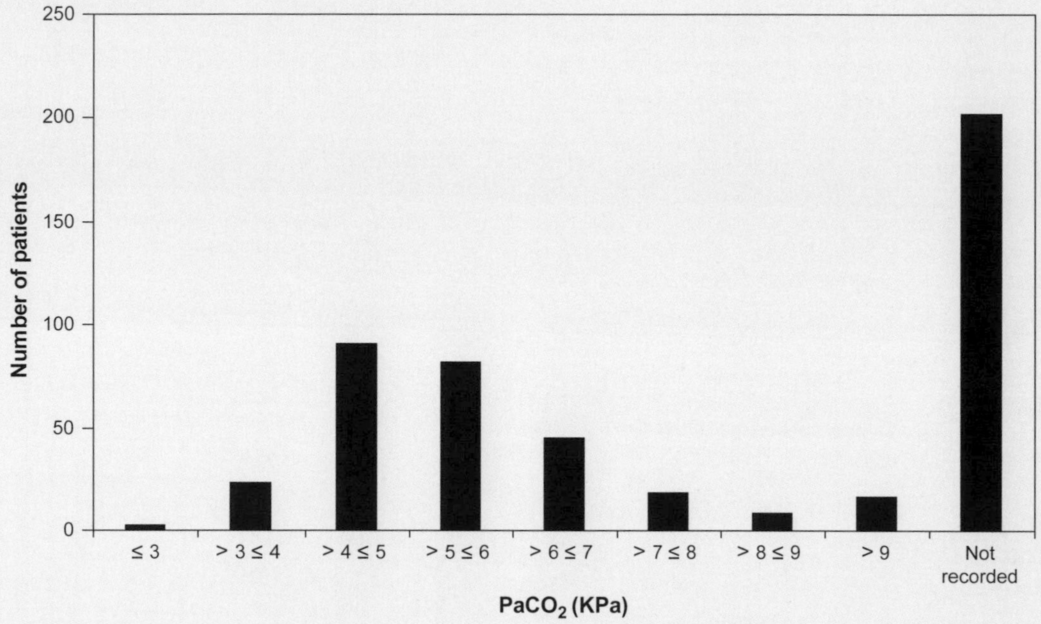

Figure 38. First documented ABG pH measurement

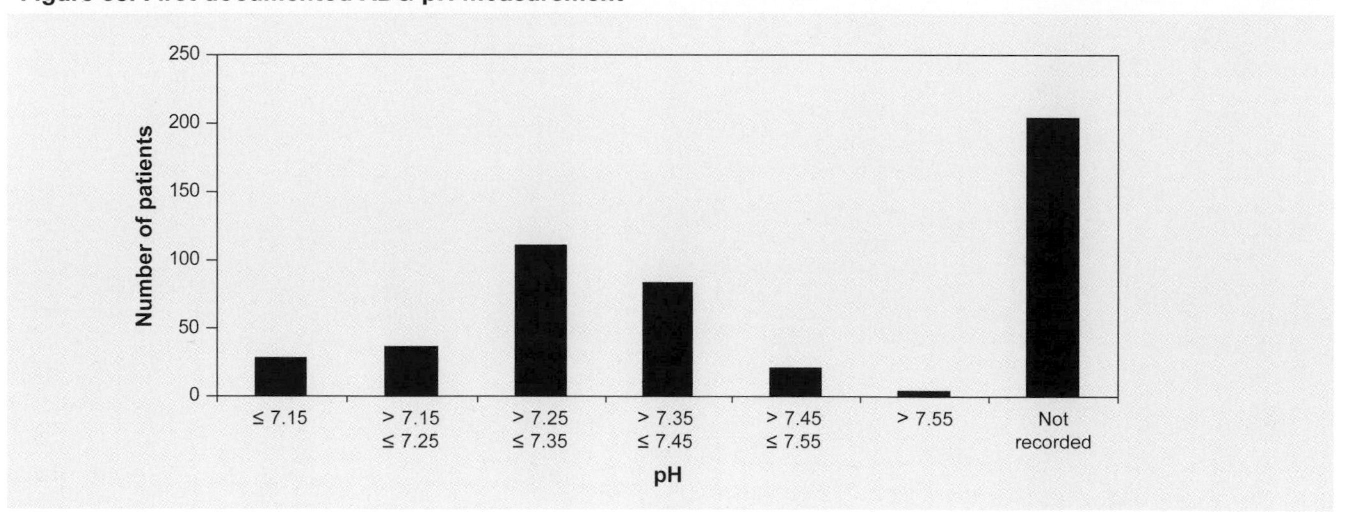

Hypoxia, hypercapnia, hypocapnia and acidosis are known to be secondary insults that can worsen outcome in the head injured patient. Hypocapnia is also detrimental to the head injured patient as it causes cerebral vasospasm and can exacerbate cerebral ischaemia. Clearly these physiological derangements are likely to occur in severely injured patients, therefore the aim of prehospital care and a well-organised emergency department response should be to minimise and rapidly correct these changes.

Given the importance of normoventilation and avoidance of both hyper and hypocapnia in the setting of traumatic brain injury the high number of patients without blood gas analysis is unacceptable.

Figure 39. Glasgow Coma Score and intubation

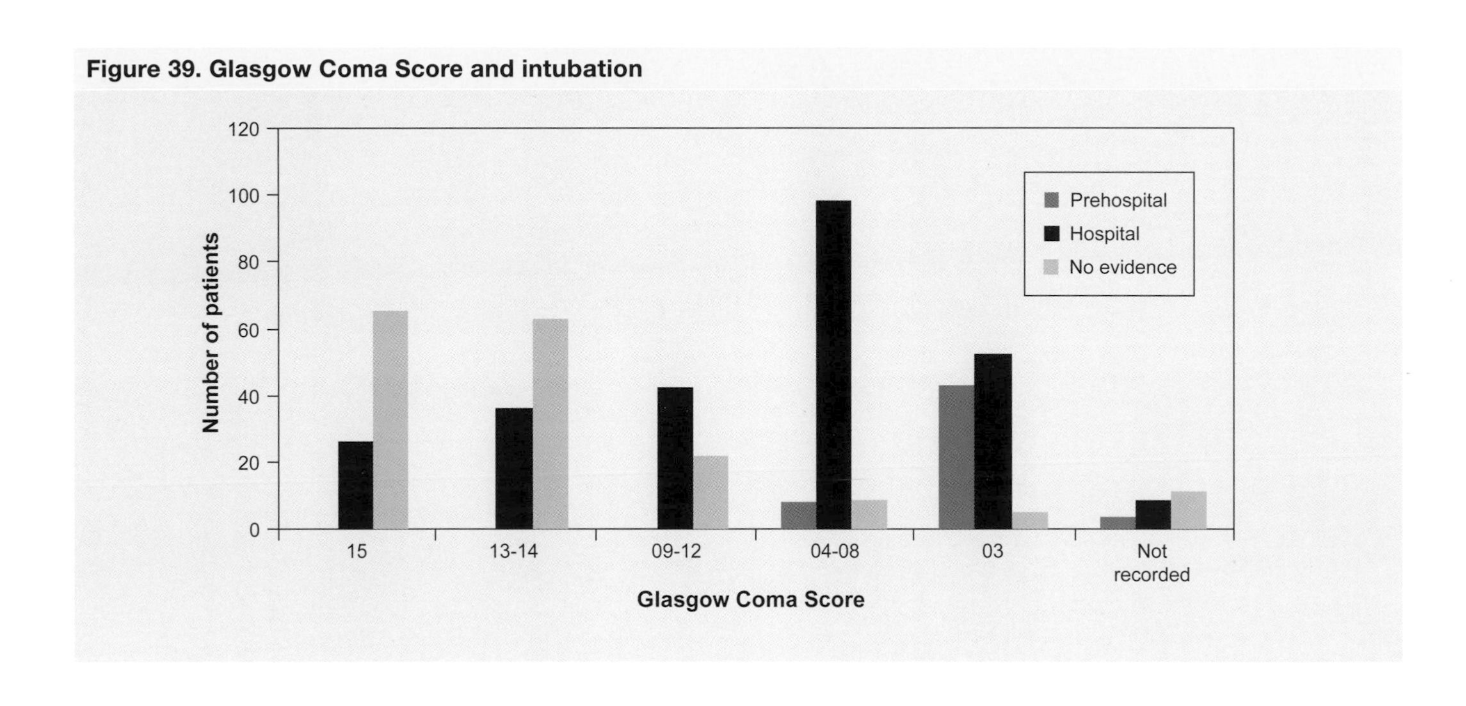

Carbon dioxide and outcome

Table 79 shows data on admission $PaCO_2$ and 72 hour mortality and illustrates the relationship between hypercapnia and poor outcome.

Table 79. $PaCO_2$ and 72 hour mortality

$PaCO_2$	Alive	Deceased	Total	Mortality (%)
≤ 3	3	0	**3**	0
> 3 ≤ 4	21	3	**24**	12.5
> 4 ≤ 5	76	15	**91**	16.5
> 5 ≤ 6	72	10	**82**	12.2
> 6 ≤ 7	37	9	**46**	19.6
> 7 ≤ 8	14	5	**19**	26.3
> 8 ≤ 9	6	3	**9**	33.3
> 9	8	9	**17**	52.9
Subtotal	**237**	**54**	**291**	**18.6**
Not recorded	169	33	**202**	16.3
Total	**406**	**87**	**493**	**17.7**

Glasgow Coma Score and intubation

Hypoxia and hypercapnia may be precipitated by problems with airway patency and/or ventilatory inadequacy. This is more likely in the group of severe head injuries (GCS <9) but can occur when there is any depression of consciousness. Intubation of the trachea and ventilatory support may be the best option to reverse these problems and prevent secondary insults. This could be performed in the prehospital setting or in the emergency department.

Figure 39 shows data about the setting of the intubation analysed by severity of head injury. In the severe head injury group, fifty one patients were intubated prehospital and another 150 patients were intubated in hospital. It should be noted that for this group (head injury), no patient with a GCS greater than 8 was intubated in the prehospital setting.

It is reasonable to assume that this group of 150 patients may have benefited from earlier intubation and hence avoidance of secondary insults. The need for prehospital intubation raises many difficult questions (who should be able to perform this task, the use of anaesthetic drugs/muscle relaxants, risk and benefits of the procedure) and these may become more relevant if the provision of services for the severely injured patient undergoes service reconfiguration. In addition it must be remembered that intubation without anaesthesia is potentially harmful to head injured patients[21].

Case study 4

A middle-aged patient was admitted to the emergency department at 22:15 hours following a fall onto the back of the head. Admission GCS was documented as 6. It appeared that the patient was admitted to the minor injuries section of the emergency department. Despite the low GCS and the history of head trauma there was no ambulance pre-alert and no trauma team response. The patient was placed in a cubical, commenced on neuro observations, given 15l/min oxygen and placed in the recovery position. No medical review happened until 23:40 when the patient was seen by an SHO. This medical review was prompted by the occurrence of a tonic-clonic seizure. The patient's GCS was recorded as 3 after this seizure. No investigation or intervention occurred at this time. The patient had a subsequent seizure at 00:05 and was given Lorazepam at that time. Finally at 01:00 the patient was taken for a CT scan. The GCS was still recorded as 3. The patient was not intubated and was escorted to radiology by the surgical SHO. The CT scan revealed a large intracerebral haemorrhage with significant midline shift. The patient was transferred back to the emergency department and at 01:30 the patient was referred to the anaesthetic SHO. The anaesthetic SHO contacted the SpR on call for anaesthesia and following their attendance the patient was intubated at 03:00. The patient subsequently died from severe brain injury.

Cerebral swelling and corticosteroids

Cerebral swelling and intracranial hypertension are other important factors in secondary brain injury. There has been a long-standing interest in the use of steroids to minimise cerebral oedema and reduce intracranial pressure. However, there are concerns over detrimental side effects caused by steroid therapy and whether, in fact, steroids confer any outcome benefit. A recent study has addressed this question[22] showing that the use of corticosteroids in traumatic brain injury caused harm. A significant increase in death and disability was found in the corticosteroid group. There was no evidence that the effect of corticosteroids differed by injury severity or time since injury. The conclusion was that corticosteroids should not be used routinely in the treatment of head injury.

There were a small number of cases (six) within this current NCEPOD study where steroids were prescribed and given to patients with head injuries as part of a management strategy to prevent brain swelling and secondary injury. Clearly this is not in line with current best evidence and cannot be supported or recommended by NCEPOD.

Investigation of head injury

The NICE guidance on management of head injuries[17] gives a list of indicators for head CT scan. The list below is taken from that guidance. Any patient who has suffered a head injury with any of these factors should have a CT scan of the head requested immediately.

Indicators for CT scanning in head injury:

GCS less than 13 on initial assessment in the emergency department,

GCS less than 15 at two hours after the injury on assessment in the emergency department,

Suspected open or depressed skull fracture,

Any sign of basal skull fracture (haemotympanum, 'panda' eyes, cerebrospinal fluid leakage from the ear or nose, Battle's sign),

Post traumatic seizure,

Focal neurological deficit,

More than one episode of vomiting,

Amnesia for events more than 30 minutes before impact.

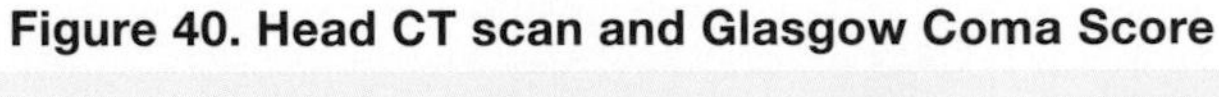

Figure 40. Head CT scan and Glasgow Coma Score

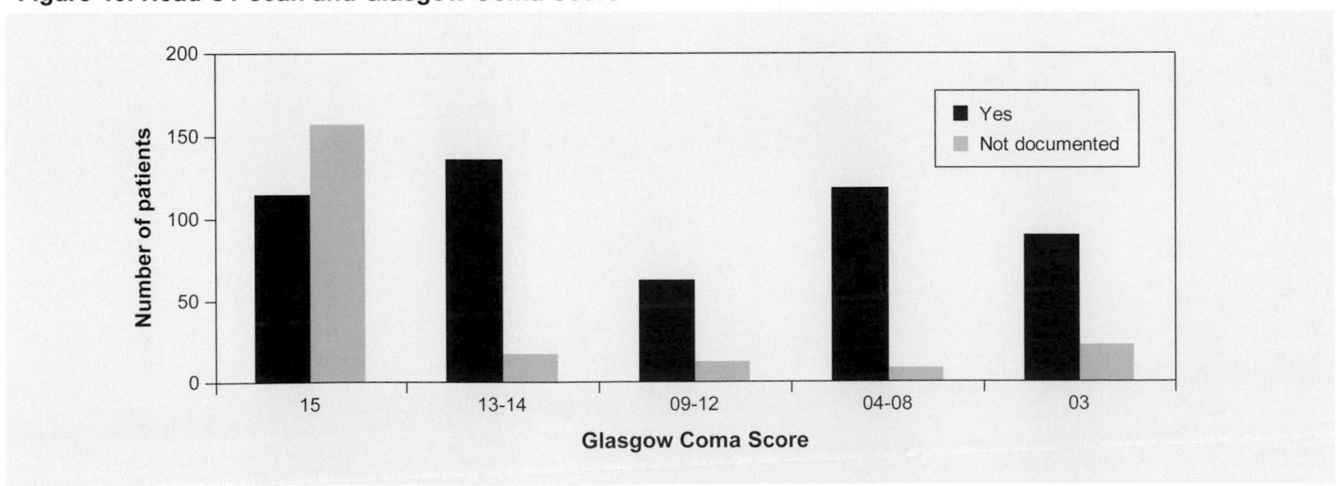

Figure 41. Time to head CT scan by Glasgow Coma Score

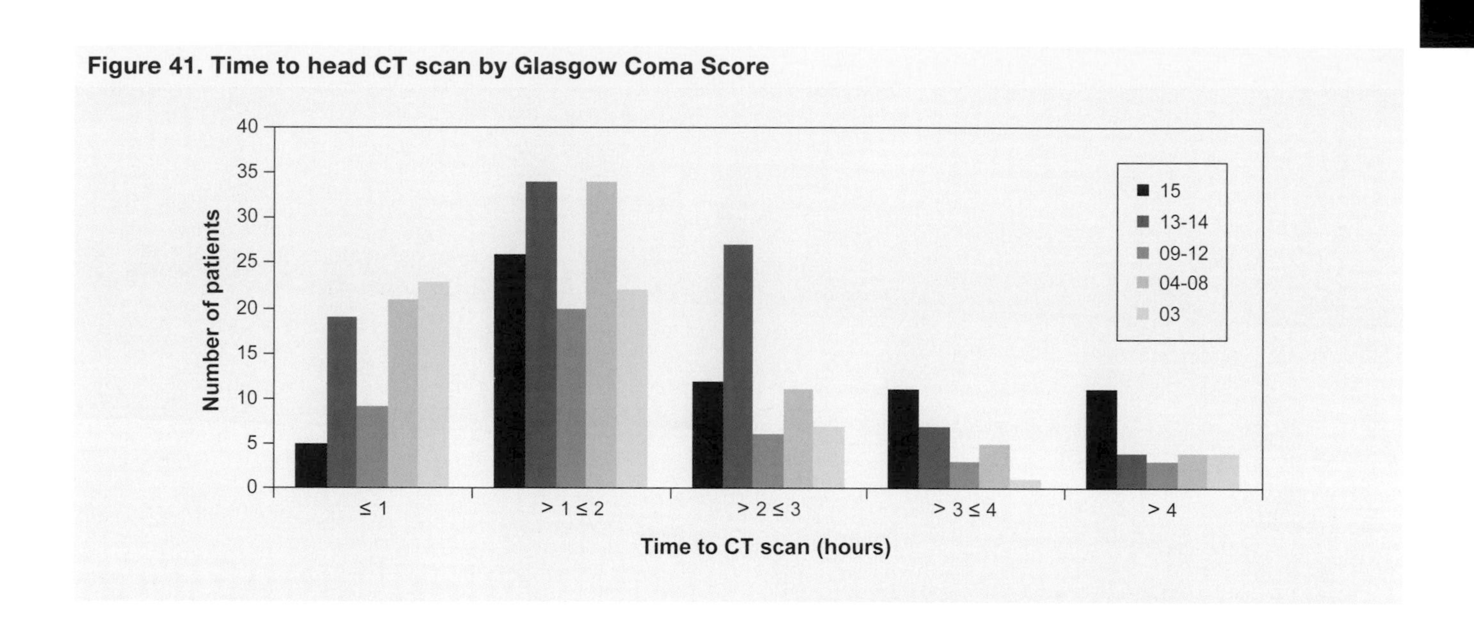

It would appear that despite this guidance some patients were not investigated appropriately. Forty-four patients with a GCS less than 13 had no evidence of head CT scanning. Without this essential investigation the scope of the injury cannot be delineated and any subsequent management plan may be sub-optimal.

Most patients who had suffered a significant head injury had a CT scan of the head (Figure 40). A small number of patients with a depressed level of consciousness did not have a CT head scan although the reasons for this decision were not clear. It may be that within the group of patients with a GCS of 3 there was no requirement for a CT head scan as the severity of the injuries led to the clinical conclusion that death was inevitable or that death occurred before CT scanning could be undertaken.

Table 80 shows the reasons, stated in the A&E clinician questionnaire, for not carrying out a CT head scan. In the majority it was felt that scanning was not clinically indicated.

Table 80. Reasons why a CT was not performed

	Number of patients	%
Not clinically indicated	128	88.9
Patient not stable enough	14	9.7
Unable to access CT	2	1.4
Subtotal	**144**	
Not answered	11	
Total	**155**	

Timing of investigation of head injury

In the event that a CT scan of the head is required, it should be performed as rapidly as possible. This does not only mean that a scan is performed in a timely fashion, but also that the images should be assessed and a report available.

Figure 41 shows the time from admission to CT scan analysed by GCS. Few scans were performed within the first hour after admission and some patients were not scanned until several hours after admission. While this may be less of a concern for patients with mild head injuries it may well be that those with moderate to severe head injuries have delays to recognition and management of remediable lesions. Unfortunately, as can be seen from Figure 41, delays to CT scanning were present across all categories of head injury severity. Thirty-two patients with severe head injuries had to wait more than two hours for this investigation to be performed.

The emergency medicine clinicians' reasons for any delays to CT head scanning are shown in Table 81.

Table 81. Reasons why there was a delay to a CT head scan

	Number of patients	%
Patient not stable	22	29.3
Awaiting radiology staff	28	37.3
Awaiting access to CT	17	22.7
Awaiting suitable medical staff	3	4.4
Other	5	6.7
Total	**75**	

The majority of cases were delayed because of organisational factors (awaiting access to CT or awaiting suitable medical staff). In only 22/75 cases was the delay considered to be due to patient instability. Again, the availability of CT radiography and radiology staff needs to be considered.

Even patient instability may be considered an organisational factor if one considers the grade of medical staff involved in the early management of these patients. As shown earlier, consultant involvement was variable (especially out of hours) and junior medical staff may be more reticent than consultants to move potentially unstable patients to the CT scanner. Furthermore, the location of the CT scanner may change the threshold for making the clinical decision that the patient is stable enough to scan; it is clearly easier and safer if the CT scanner is close to the emergency department rather than in a remote area.

NICE gives guidance on the timing of CT scan after head injury[17]. The guidance states that in those circumstances described earlier:

Figure 42. Timeliness of CT scan by Glasgow Coma Score (advisors' opinion)

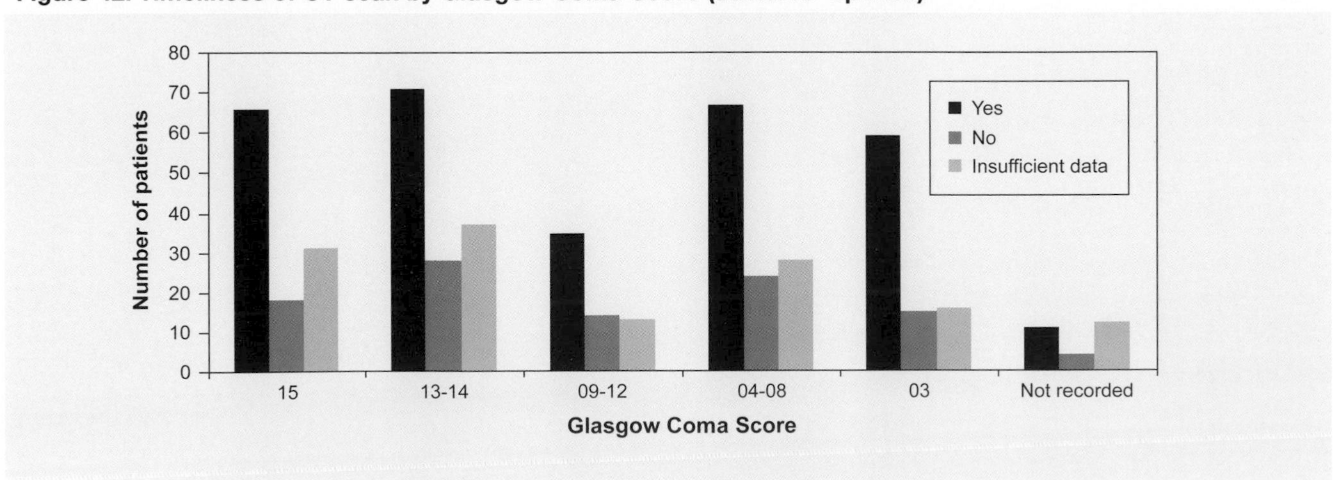

"CT imaging of the head should be performed (i.e. imaging carried out and results analysed) within one hour of the request having been received by the radiology department."

The practice demonstrated in this dataset fell well short of that guidance. As a result there is the potential for delays in both diagnosis and subsequent management of reversible pathology.

Advisor assessment of investigation of head injury

The advisors assessed whether a head CT scan was a necessary part of each patient's management. Table 82 shows these data and makes the point that there was general agreement between the clinical decisions and the advisors' opinions. However, in 23/539 cases it was thought that a CT scan was performed unnecessarily. Also in 24/220 cases a CT scan was indicated although this was not performed: and it was felt that the lack of CT scanning may have missed potentially treatable pathology.

Table 82. Advisors' opinion on the necessity of a head CT scan

	CT necessary				
CT scan	**Yes**	**No**	**Subtotal**	**Insufficient data**	**Total**
Yes	516	23	**539**	10	**549**
No	24	196	**220**	26	**246**
Total	**540**	**219**	**759**	**36**	**795**

In addition to the need for CT scanning, the advisors were also asked to consider whether this was performed in a timely fashion. Figure 42 shows this opinion analysed by severity of head injury. Overall, the advisors believed that one in four CT scans (103/412) were not performed in a timely fashion. Patients with severe head injuries, whose management is most time critical, did not appear to have more timely investigations. Again it should be noted that the main reasons for delay were organisational, rather than patient related, factors.

Interpretation of CT scans

Accurate interpretation of the CT scan is essential. Tables 83 and 84 show the grade and specialty of clinicians involved. The majority of images were reported by consultant radiologists. These data were taken from the A&E questionnaire and most likely reflect the final report of the CT scan. Most investigations performed, particularly out of hours, had a provisional report written in the notes by a more junior doctor.

Table 83. Grade of clinician interpreting the CT scan

	Number of patients	%
Consultant	196	59.9
NCCG	1	<1
SpR	37	11.3
SpR1/2	7	2.1
SpR3	85	26.0
SHO	1	<1
Subtotal	**327**	
Not answered	24	
Total	**351**	

Table 84. The specialty of the clinician interpreting the CT scan

	Number of patients	%
Radiology	312	94.8
Emergency medicine	10	3.0
Neurology	6	1.8
Anaesthetics	1	<1
Subtotal	**329**	
Not answered	22	
Total	**351**	

Neurosurgical and neurocritical care

The need for neurosurgeons to take a leadership role in developing local guidelines and protocols for head injury was highlighted in a recent report from the Royal College of Surgeons of England[23]. In most instances, patients with severe head injury have to be transferred to a neurosurgical unit. Since the time from injury to evacuation of an intracranial haematoma is critical for a good outcome (four hours is considered the maximum permissible delay), all components of the healthcare system must operate smoothly. Hospitals accepting patients with head injuries should have 24 hour facilities for CT scanning, with an image link facility to the regional neurosurgical unit. Although rapid transfer is important, it should not compromise basic resuscitation and restoration of physiological stability. Furthermore, the organisation of the referral and subsequent transfer should not compromise ongoing clinical management. Standards for transfer of such patients have been laid out in guidelines that stress the importance of experienced anaesthetic staff travelling with the patient and avoiding hypotension and hypoxia during transfer[24].

Neurosurgical consultation

Many trauma patients who have suffered a head injury are initially taken to non-neurosurgical centres. A key part of the management of these patients is close collaboration with the regional neurosurgical service. Often this collaboration occurs when a CT scan has been performed and the images and case are discussed by the receiving clinician and the neurosurgical service.

Figure 43. Neurosurgeon consulted by Glasgow Coma Score

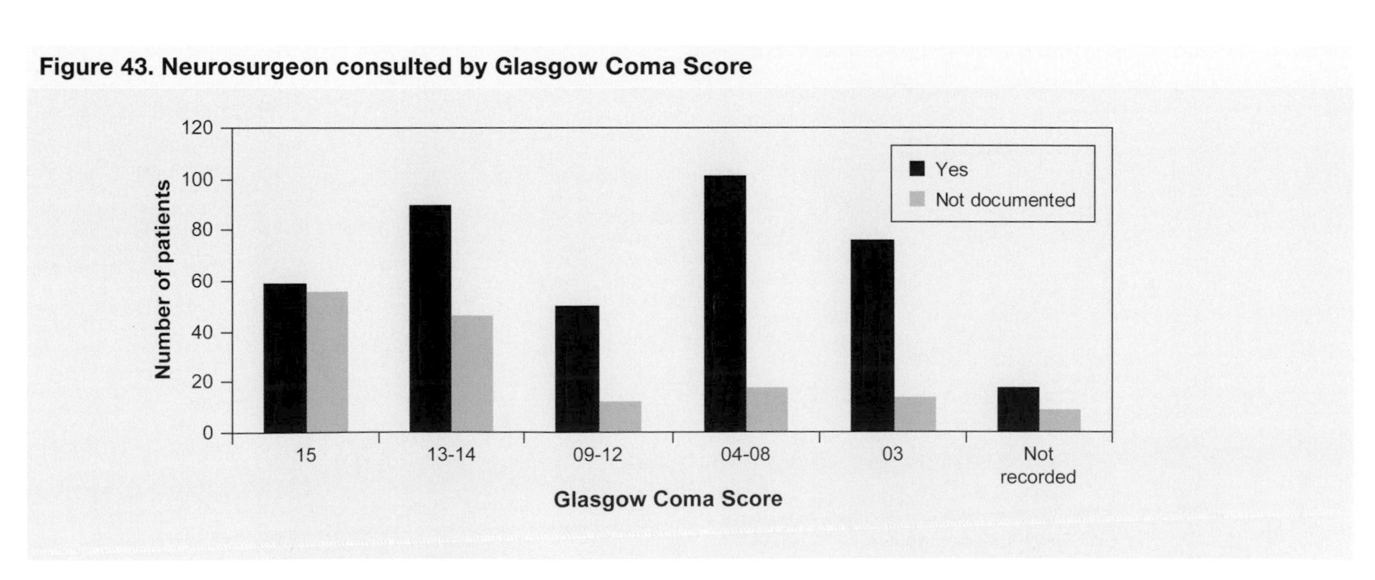

Figure 44. Location of consulted neurosurgeon

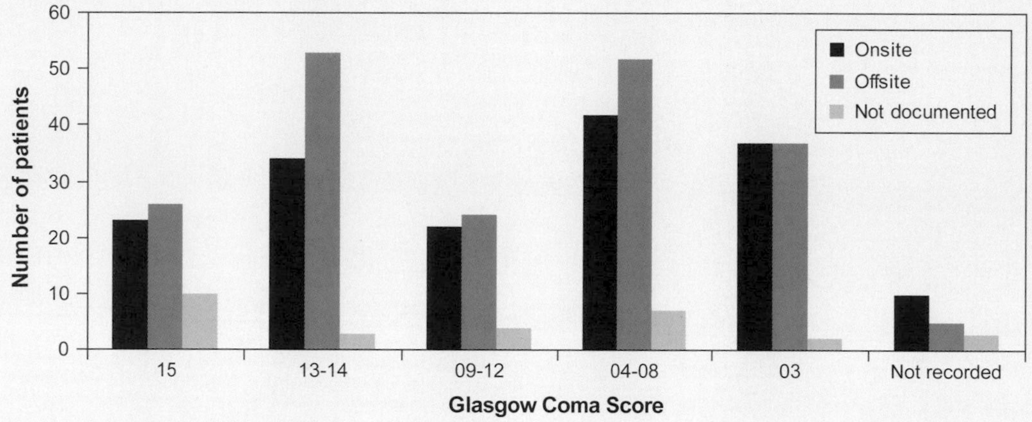

Figure 43 shows data on whether there was discussion with the neurosurgical service. In the majority of cases where a patient suffered a head injury, a neurosurgical consultation was performed. However, it was noted that 44/271 (16.2%) patients with moderate or severe head injuries had no evidence of neurosurgical involvement. Within this group of 44 patients it is possible that consultation was not undertaken due to the extent of head and/or other injuries leading to the conclusion that death was inevitable.

As part of the peer review process, advisors were asked whether a neurosurgical consultation was a necessary part of each individual case. Of the 155 cases where there was no evidence of neurosurgical involvement the advisors felt that this should have occurred in 28 cases (18.1%).

Location of neurosurgical support

Figure 44 shows the location of the neurosurgical service in relation to the admission location. More patients received offsite neurosurgical support than onsite.

These data suggest that 197/365 (54.0%) patients who required neurosurgical involvement were taken to hospitals that may not have had the necessary infrastructure (on site neurosurgical expertise) to meet their needs. Given the time critical nature of neurosurgical intervention in traumatic brain injury this had the potential to introduce delays into definitive management, which may affect outcome. Although we accept that in many circumstances taking the patient directly to a neurosurgical centre may be more appropriate, consideration of the pattern and severity of injuries and the likely services required should be taken into account when the prehospital clinicians are transporting the severely injured patient to hospital. However, it does appear that direct admission to a trauma centre compared to secondary transfer is associated with a better outcome[25] and neurosurgeons and ambulance trusts should agree protocols on this aspect of care.

Time to neurosurgical consultation

The availability of onsite neurosurgical support may affect time to consultation and intervention. In 14 cases it was not known if the consultation was on or offsite. These data are shown in Table 85.

Table 85. Time (hours) to neurosurgical consultation

	All	(%)	Onsite	(%)	Offsite	(%)
≤ 1	26	10.2	15	13.6	8	6.2
>1≤2	56	22.1	24	21.8	30	23.1
>2≤3	54	21.3	20	18.2	30	23.1
>3≤4	32	12.6	7	6.4	24	18.5
>4≤5	21	8.3	5	4.6	7	5.4
>5≤6	14	5.5	13	11.8	8	6.2
>6≤12	28	11.0	10	9.1	17	13.1
>12	23	9.1	16	14.6	6	4.6
Total	**254**		**110**		**130**	

Neurocritical care capacity

The supply of emergency neurosurgical beds in the UK is limited. A recent survey revealed that only 43 neurosurgical intensive care beds are available for an overall estimated population of 63.6 million[26]. This shortfall can lead to delays in patient transfer, and is symptomatic of larger resource and workload issues for neurosurgery in the UK[27]. These larger resource problems have many implications for head injury care, including delays obtaining a neurosurgical opinion at night, or at the weekend.

One consequence of this lack of capacity in neurosurgical critical care beds is that some patients may stay in their 'local' critical care unit rather than be transferred to the neurosurgical centre. This may have an adverse effect on patient outcome. In a recent study it was shown that patients with severe head injury who were treated only in non-neurosurgical centres had a 26% increase in mortality and a 2.15-fold increase (95% CI 1.77-2.60) in the odds of death adjusted for case mix compared with patients treated at a neurosurgical centre[28]. This suggests that transfer to, and treatment in, a neurosurgical centre is an important part of the management plan for patients with severe head injury.

Case study 5

A young patient was admitted to hospital after sustaining a head injury. Admission GCS was 5. CT head scanning revealed a large intracerebral haemorrhage, cerebral oedema and midline shift. Referral was made to the regional neurosurgical centre at 01:15. The neurosurgical SpR stated that there were no beds in the ICU and advised that the patient be referred to another neurosurgical centre. After some difficulty in contacting the on call neurosurgeon, the patient was discussed with the neurosurgical SpR at a second centre. This occurred at 02:15. The neurosurgical SpR stated that they had beds available and would be prepared to take the patient but that the opinion of whether transfer should occur should be made by the local neurosurgical centre that had no capacity to take the patient. A further telephone call was made to the local neurosurgical centre at 02:30 who felt that as they had no capacity they could not comment on the patient care. At 03:00 a second telephone call was made to the second neurosurgical centre and at that point the neurosurgical SpR requested that hard copies of the CT be sent to him. Six more telephone calls occurred over the next few hours between the initial hospital and three different neurosurgical centres. By 06:30 the patient, who was still in the emergency department, had fixed and dilated pupils and it was believed that death was the inevitable outcome. The patient was admitted to ICU and after a period of family discussion ventilatory support was withdrawn. At no time was brain stem death confirmed or considered. Organ donation, either heart beating or non-heart beating, was never discussed.

Within this current study there were many, albeit less extreme, instances of difficulties in contacting the neurosurgeon on call, lack of willingness to accept patients with severe head injuries, lack of capacity in neurosurgical centres and clear lack of protocols to smooth the process of care between the local centres and the neurosurgical centre.

Neurosurgical procedures

The number of patients who undergo major neurosurgical procedures each year following a head injury is also unclear. A figure of around 4,000 patients per year for the UK as a whole has been quoted[29], but this may an overestimate. Hospital Episode Statistics data for the 2000/2001 annual dataset indicate that 398 patients in England underwent an operation to drain the extradural space (OPCS code A40) and 2,048 patients underwent an operation to drain the subdural space (OPCS code A41)[30]. These figures do not include a number of other neurosurgical procedures possible after head injury (including burr hole for chronic subdural haematoma or insertion of intracranial pressure monitors), and include some patients with a non-head injury diagnosis. Thus, the routine data available does not allow for a precise figure of neurosurgical volume after head injury for England and Wales, but points to a figure in the low thousands.

Table 86. Type of surgery performed

	Number of patients	%
Evacuation of subdural haematoma	20	17.5
Evacuation of extradural haematoma	22	19.3
Evacuation of intracerebral haematoma / contusion	7	6.1
Insertion of intracranial pressure bolt only	48	42.1
Elevation of fracture	7	6.1
Decompressive craniectomy	5	4.4
Other	5	4.4
Total	**114**	

Table 86 shows that 114 patients had a surgical procedure as a consequence of head trauma (23% of the head injured patients). The majority of this activity (48 cases) involved the insertion of an intracranial pressure (ICP) monitoring device, with no further surgery in the first 72 hours. A further 54 operations were related to the evacuation of traumatic space occupying lesions or decompressive craniectomy.

Grade of operating surgeon

Table 87 shows the grade of clinician performing the surgery. Only 15.8% of interventions were documented as being performed by consultants.

Table 87. Grade of surgeon performing the surgery

	Number of patients	%
Consultant	12	15.8
SpR	56	73.7
SHO	8	10.5
Subtotal	76	
Not documented	38	
Total	**114**	

This was a lower level of consultant involvement than has been seen in past NCEPOD studies[31,32]. Given the volume of surgery performed annually as a result of head trauma[29] this potentially represents a substantial amount of surgery performed by doctors in training. However, the insertion of an intracranial pressure monitor is generally performed at the bedside and is likely to be an appropriate procedure to be delegated to junior neurosurgical staff with sufficient training.

For this reason Table 88 shows the grade of surgeon for the cases excluding insertion of an ICP monitor.

Table 88. Grade of surgeon excluding insertion of an ICP monitor

	Number of patients	%
Consultant	9	18.8
SpR	38	79.2
SHO	1	2.1
Subtotal	**48**	
Not recorded	18	
Total	**66**	

Even when these more minor procedures have been excluded only 18.8% (9/48) of operations were documented as being performed by a consultant.

During expert and advisor group meetings to discuss the findings in this study the issue of consultant neurosurgical involvement generated significant discussion. Whilst the insertion of an intracranial pressure monitor may well be within the remit of appropriately trained junior staff, most major neurosurgical procedures were being performed by these same staff in training.

The system of junior staff care is also changing: European Working Time Directive, Modernising Medical Careers and the Hospital at Night project have significantly changed the level of junior staff experience and support from that available in previous years.

Given this discussion, it is felt that the low level of direct consultant involvement in the management of patients who require major neurosurgical procedures is undesirable and that a much higher input is required.

Time to neurosurgical intervention

Table 89 shows time to surgery analysed by whether the patient required a secondary transfer to another site to have this surgery performed.

Table 89. Time to surgery (hours)

	Onsite		Transferred	
		%		%
≤ 4	22	66.7	6	14.0
>4 ≤ 8	9	27.3	23	53.5
>8 ≤ 12	2	6.0	4	9.3
>12	0	0	10	23.3
Subtotal	**33**		**43**	
Not recorded	23		15	
Total	**56**		**58**	

The requirement for a secondary transfer significantly increased the time to surgical intervention. Indeed, only 6/43 patients requiring transfer had neurosurgery within the first four hours after injury. Intensive head injury care begins at the scene of the accident. It includes protecting the airway and cerebral circulation which may involve the urgent removal of clots, but may also (or only) require the insertion of pressure monitors to guide longer-term therapy. Rapid surgery is crucial for patients with intracerebral haematomas requiring evacuation, where every moment's delay jeopardises eventual outcome, but is less vital for patients requiring intracerebral pressure monitoring as part of the overall intensive care management of diffuse brain injury. For this reason, despite surgery occurring after four hours in 11/33 (33.3%) of onsite patients and 37/43 (86.0%) of transferred patients, these operations were considered timely in 68/81 (84.0%). Of the 16% of cases where it was felt that surgery was not performed in a timely manner, 10/13 required evacuation of clots or craniectomies where delays are undesirable and have a negative impact on outcome (Table 90).

This delay is in keeping with a recent study which showed that the mean transfer time to a neurosurgical centre for patients with an extradural haematoma and subdural haematoma was 5.25 and 6 hours respectively[33].

Clearly these delays may affect outcome and this again raises the issue of transfer to an appropriate hospital in the first instance and reconfiguration of trauma services for regions.

Table 90. Timeliness of neurosurgery

	Number of patients	%
Yes	68	84.0
No	13	16.0
Subtotal	**81**	
Insufficient data	33	
Total	**114**	

Overall assessment of management of head injured patients

The advisors were asked to assess the overall management of the patient using the grading system detailed in the methods section (Table 91).

Table 91. Overall assessment of head injury management

	Number of patients	
		%
Good practice	205	41.6
Room for improvement clinical	80	16.2
Room for improvement organisational	114	23.1
Room for improvement clinical and organisational	46	9.3
Less than satisfactory	25	5.1
Insufficient data	23	4.7
Total	**493**	

Less than half the patients (205/493) were thought to have received a standard of care that could be described as good practice. In 240/493 (48.7%) cases it was thought that there was room for improvement in organisational and /or clinical aspects of care. Of concern were the 25/493 (5.1%) cases where it was thought that patient management was less than satisfactory, signifying a significant problem in the care process.

Key findings

Head trauma is very common in the severely injured patient and has a negative impact on outcome.

Secondary insults (hypoxia, hypercapnia and hypotension) are common and these are known to worsen eventual outcome (higher mortality and more severe disability).

The prehospital management of the airway and ventilation was inadequate in 14.3% and 10.6% of cases respectively.

In a small number of cases steroids are being used in the routine management of the head injured patient, despite evidence that this therapy may cause harm.

One in five patients who required a head CT scan did not have this performed in a timely fashion.

Delays in CT scanning were primarily due to organisational factors rather than patient factors.

More than half of the patients who required neurosurgical advice or input were taken to hospitals where there was no onsite neurosurgical service.

Only 6/43 (14.0%) patients who required a secondary transfer to access neurosurgical services had an operation within four hours of injury.

There were delays to neurosurgery in 13/81 (16.0%) cases. Most of these cases were evacuation of traumatic space occupying lesions.

Only 9/48 (18.8%) patients who had major neurosurgical procedures as a result of trauma were operated on by consultant surgeons.

Less than half of the severely injured patients who suffered head trauma received a standard of care that was judged to be good practice.

Recommendations

Prehospital assessment of neurological status should be performed in all cases where head injury is apparent or suspected. This should be performed using the Glasgow Coma Scale. Pupil size and reactivity should also be recorded. *(Ambulance trusts)*

A pre-alert should be made for all trauma patients with a GCS less than or equal to 8, to ensure appropriately experienced professionals are available for their treatment and to prepare for imaging. *(Ambulance trusts)*

Patients with severe head injury require early definitive airway control and rapid delivery to a centre with onsite neurosurgical service. This implies regional planning of trauma services, including prehospital physician involvement, and reconfiguration of services. *(Ambulance and hospital trusts)*

Patients with severe head injury should have a CT head scan performed as soon as possible after admission and within one hour of arrival at hospital. *(Trauma team leader and radiology heads)*

All patients with moderate or severe head injury should have case and CT findings discussed with a neurosurgical service. *(Trauma team lead)*

All patients with severe head injury should be transferred to a neurosurgical/critical care centre irrespective of the requirement for surgical intervention. *(Strategic health authorities, hospital trusts, trauma team leaders)*

Consultant presence should be increased at operations requiring major neurosurgery. *(Hospital trusts)*

References

1. Teasdale GH. J Neurol Neurosurg Psychiatry 1995; 58: 855-887

2. Rose J, Valtonen S, Jennett B. *Avoidable factors contributing to death after head injury.* BMJ 1977; 2: 615-8

3. Jennett B, Carlin J. *Preventable mortality and morbidity after head injury.* Injury 1978; 10: 31-9

4. Rockswold GL, Leonard PR, Nagib MG. *Analysis of management in thirty-three closed head injury patients who 'talked and deteriorated'.* Neurosurgery 1987; 21: 51-5

5. Mendelow AD, Karma MZ, Paul KS, Fuller GA, Gillingham FJ. *Extradural haematoma: effect of delayed treatment.* BMJ 1979; I: 1240-2

6. Klauber MR, Marshall LF, Luerssen TG, Frankowski R, Tabaddor K, Eisenberg HM. *Determinants of head injury mortality: importance of the low risk patient.* Neurosurgery 1989; 24: 31-6

7. O'Sullivan MG, Gray WP, Buckley TF. *Extradural haematoma in the Irish Republic: an analysis of 82 cases with emphasis on delay.* Br J Surg 1990; 77: 1391-4

8. Brain Trauma Foundation, American Association of Neurological Surgeons, Joint Section on Neurotrauma and Critical Care. Guidelines for the management of severe head injury. J. Neurotrauma 1996; 13: 641-734

9. The management of acute head injury: seminar papers. London: DHSS 1983

10. Guidelines for initial management after head injury in adults. Suggestions from a group of neurosurgeons. BMJ 1984 288: 983-5

11. Report of the Working Party on Head Injuries. London: Royal College of Surgeons of England Commission on the Provision of Surgical Services; 1986

12. Bartlett J, Kett-White R, Mendelow AD, Miller JD, Pickard J, Teasdale G. *Recommendations from the Society of British Neurological Surgeons.* Br J Neurosurg 1998; 12(4): 349-52

13. The Royal College of Radiologists. Making the best use of a department of clinical radiology: guidelines for Doctors. 4th Ed. London; The College; 1998

14. Royal College of Surgeons of England. Report of the Working Party on the Management of Patients with Head Injuries. London: The College; 1999

15. Working Party of the British Paediatric Association and British Association of Paediatric Surgeons, Joint Standing Committee in Childhood Accidents. Guidelines on the Management of Head Injuries in Childhood. London: British Paediatric Association; 1991

16. Scottish Intercollegiate Guidelines Network: Early Management of Patients with a head injury. 2007. – *http://www.sign.ac.uk/guidelines/fulltext/46/index.html*

17. National Institute for Health and Clinical Excellence. Managing head injury: updated NICE guidelines.2007. – *http://www.nice.org.uk/page.aspx?o=455350*

18. Chi JH, Knudson MM, Vassar MJ, et al. *Prehospital hypoxia affects outcome in patients with traumatic brain injury: a prospective multicenter study.* J Trauma. 2006 Nov; 61(5):1134-41

19. Brain Trauma Foundation, American Association of Neurological Surgeons, Joint Section on Neurotrauma and Critical Care. Guidelines for the management of severe head injury. J. Neurotrauma 1996; 13: 641-734

20. Chestnut RM, Marshall LF, Klauber MR et al. *The role of secondary brain injury in determining outcome from severe head injury.* J Trauma. 1993; 34(2):216-22

21. Dunham CM, Barraco RD, Clark DE, et al.; *EAST Practice Management Guidelines Work Group. Guidelines for emergency tracheal intubation immediately after traumatic injury.* J Trauma 2003; 55:162-197

22. Edwards P, Arango M, Balica L, et al. *CRASH trial collaborators. Final results of MRC CRASH, a randomised placebo-controlled trial of intravenous corticosteroid in adults with head injury-outcomes at 6 months.* Lancet. 2005; 365(9475):1957-9

23. The Royal College of Surgeons of England. Report of the working party on the management of head injuries. London: RCS, 1999

24. Working party of the Neuroanaesthesia Society and Association of Anaesthetists. Recommendations for the transfer of patients with acute head injuries to neurosurgical units. Neuroanaesthesia Society of Great Britain and Ireland and the Association of Anaesthetists of Great Britain and Ireland, 1996

25. Sampalis JS, Denis R, Fréchette P, Brown R, Fleiszer D, Mulder D. *Direct transport to tertiary trauma centers versus transfer from lower level facilities: impact on mortality and morbidity among patients with major trauma.* 1997 Aug;43(2):288-295

26. Crimmins DW, Palmer JD. *Snapshot view of emergency neurosurgical head injury care in Great Britain and Ireland.* J Neurol Neurosurg Psychiatry 2000; 68: 8-13

27. Ashkan K, Edwards RJ, Bell BA. *Crisis in resources: a neurosurgical perspective.* Br J Neurosurg 2001; 15: 342-6

28. Patel HC, Bouamra O, Woodford M, King AT, Yates DW, Lecky FE. *Trends in head injury outcome from 1989 to 2003 and the effect of neurosurgical care: an observational study.* Lancet. 2005; 29-Nov 4;366(9496):1538-44

29. Safe Neurosurgery 2000. A Report from the Society of British Neurological Surgeons. Nelson MJ, SBNS, 35-43 Lincoln's Inn Fields, London

30. Hospital Episode Statistics. 2000/2001. Department of Health

31. *Abdominal Aortic Aneurysm: A service in need of surgery?* National Confidential Enquiry into Patient Outcome and Death. 2005. *http://www.ncepod.org.uk*

32. *Who Operates When II?* National Confidential Enquiry into Patient Outcome and Death. 2005. *http://www.ncepod.org.uk*

33. Leach P, Childs C, Evans J, Johnston N, Protheroe R, King A.*Transfer times for patients with extradural and subdural haematomas to neurosurgery in Greater Manchester.* Br J Neurosurg. 2007 Feb; 21(1):11-5

CHAPTER 9 - Paediatric care

Organisational data

Injury remains a leading cause of death in childhood. In the UK three million children present to emergency departments each year following injury. The majority of attendances at emergency departments are due to moderate or minor injuries. The absolute numbers of severe injuries are low and these patients present to a number of different hospitals. Therefore it is more difficult to maintain specific clinical skills in the management of severe trauma in children.

The injuries sustained by children differ from those of adults and consequently there are significant differences in their post-trauma management. In particular, the incidence of head trauma is more common in the paediatric population.

The definitions of neonates, infants and children differed between hospitals. The maximum age of a neonate as defined by the departments surveyed varied between 1 and 24 months. The maximum age of infants varied from 12 to 60 months. Two thirds of departments (110/183; 60.1%)

Figure 45. Availability of an advanced paediatric life support provider resident or 24 hours a day

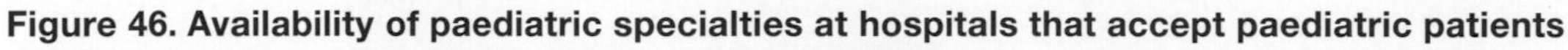

Figure 46. Availability of paediatric specialties at hospitals that accept paediatric patients

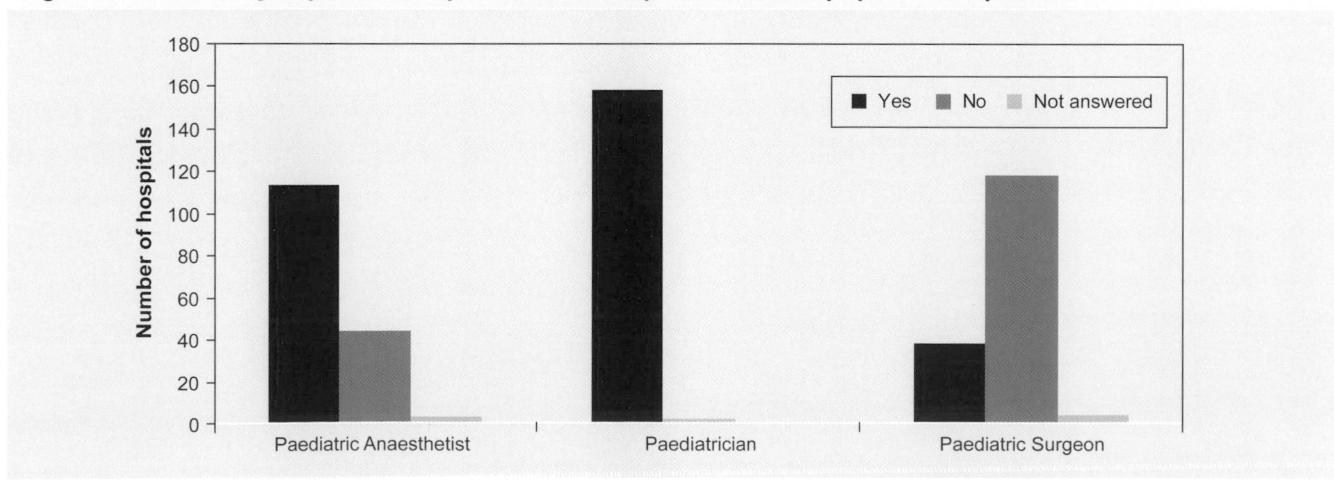

defined children as being up to 16 years of age, but 9.8% (18/183) had a higher maximum age; the oldest being 19 years of age.

An Advanced Paediatric Life Support (APLS) provider was resident or available 24 hours a day in 79.8% of hospitals (Figure 45).

Protocols

It is recommended that protocols for the management of paediatric cases should be in place[1]. One hundred and fifty five (84.7%) of the 183 sites for which an organisational questionnaire was returned to NCEPOD had up to date guidelines for the management of paediatric trauma. Of the 160 hospitals (87.4%) which accepted children for definitive care, 23 (14.4%) did not have up to date guidelines for the management of children.

Thirteen out of 22 (59.1%) sites that did not admit children for definitive care had a bypass protocol in place in order to reduce the likelihood of a severely injured child being brought to the hospital.

If non-accidental injury is suspected in children, up to date guidelines on the management and referral of these patients should be in place. One hundred and seventy six (96.2%) hospitals had up to date guidelines on referral and management of suspected non-accidental injury in children.

Facilities and staffing in hospitals accepting children for definitive care

It was recommended in the Better Care for the Severely Injured Patient Report[2] that "any hospital receiving and caring for the severely injured child must have on-site support from paediatrics' and paediatric anaesthetists".

As Figure 46 illustrates, the majority of hospitals accepting paediatric patients had a specialist in paediatric anaesthesia and a consultant paediatrician; 70.6% (113/160) and 98.8% (158/160) respectively. Guidelines do not specify the need for a paediatric surgical consultant at all hospitals accepting children. Only 23.8% (38/160) of hospitals accepting children for definitive care have a paediatric surgical consultant, suggesting that the transfer of patients to these sites for surgery is often necessary.

The Royal College of Surgeons of England guidelines also recommend that hospitals admitting children have a full range of appropriate resuscitation equipment[2]. Of the emergency departments at these hospitals 149/160 (93.2%) had a listed and checked mobile equipment kit to assist in the resuscitation of children.

It is recommended that emergency departments receiving children should have a children's nurse available at all times. A Registered Sick Children's Nurse (RSCN) was available at 146/160 (91.3%) of hospitals accepting children. However, only 22 of these 146 hospitals (15.1%) had cover 24 hours a day, 7 days a week.

Clearly there are difficulties in providing all necessary staff for the comprehensive management of the paediatric trauma patient. The data above shows problems with paediatric anaesthetic support and paediatric surgical support in some centres. This is in the context of the centralisation of many specialised paediatric services including surgery, neurosurgery and paediatric intensive care medicine. Some hospitals have acknowledged this fact by the use of protocols to avoid admitting severely injured children. The use of such protocols and close working within a network to provide trauma care to children is required.

Clinical data

Age range

There were 68 patients included in the study who were aged 16 years of age or less.

Most of the data analyses in the previous chapters were repeated for this small subset of patients. Only in a very few cases did the analysis show any different patterns from the whole sample. The bulk of this report is therefore applicable to both adults and children and the analysis will not be presented again for this group.

Figure 47. Age range of patient sample

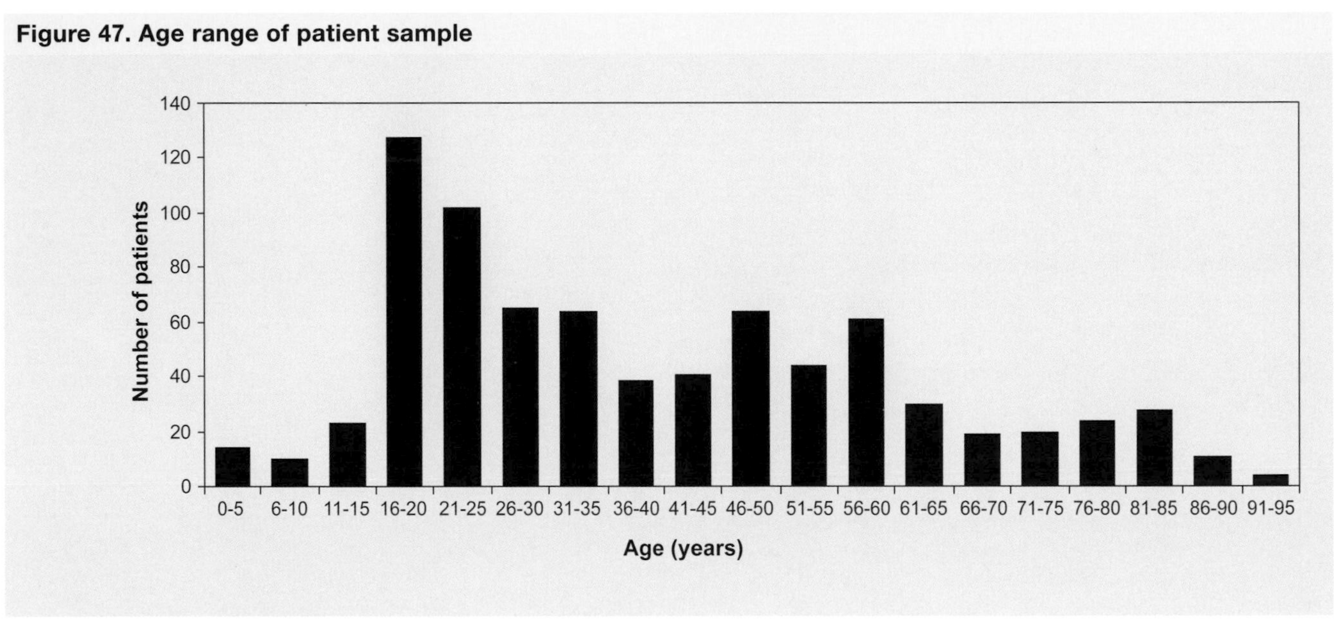

Figure 48. Overall assessment of care (advisors' view)

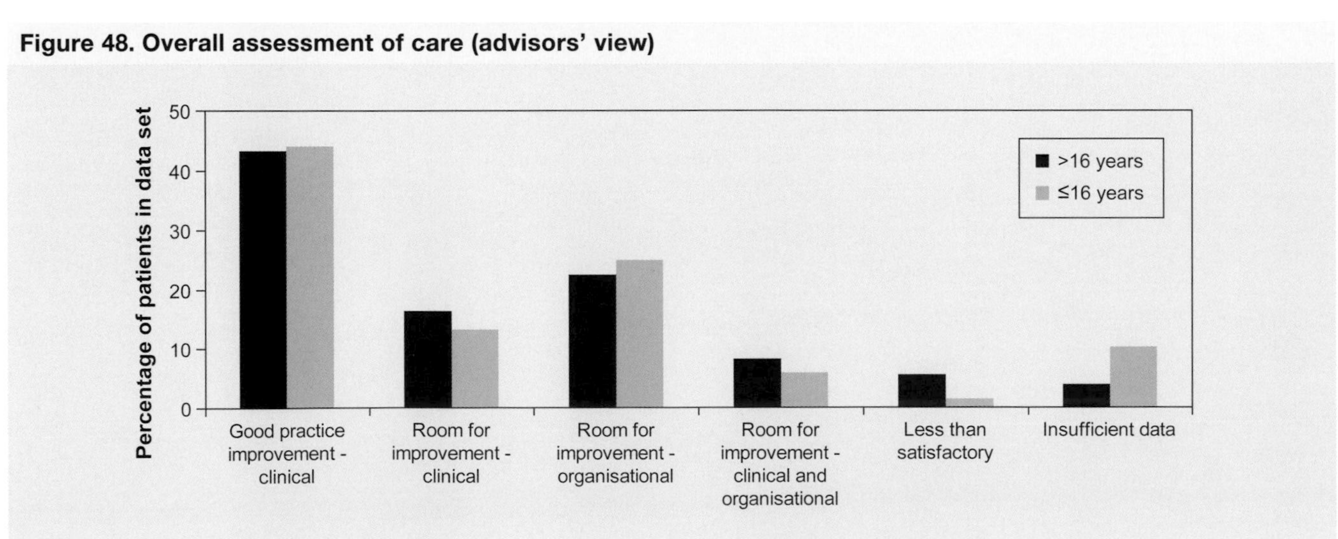

Figure 49. Grade of first reviewer/team leader

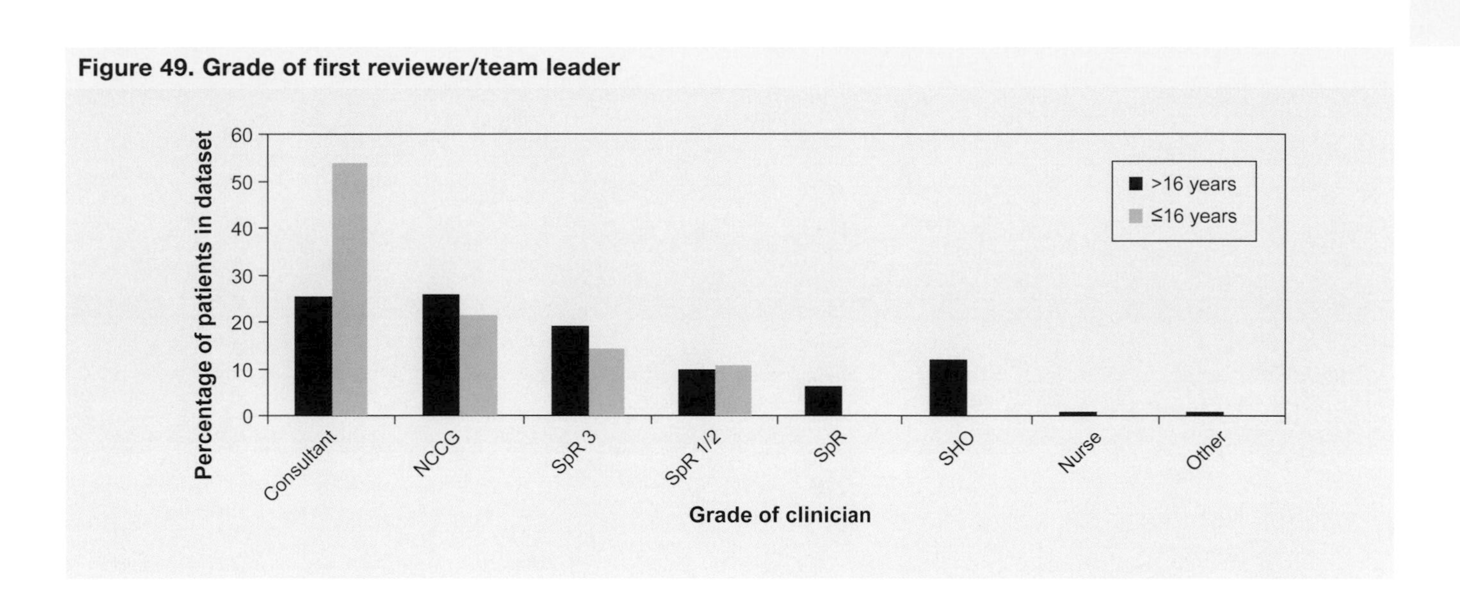

Overall assessment of care

Figure 48 shows overall assessment of care for the paediatric sample compared with the adult sample. There was little difference between the two groups.

Grade of first reviewer/team leader

Figure 49 shows grade of first reviewer/team leader analysed by age of patient. In comparison with the adult data, it was encouraging that there was more consultant involvement in the initial management, but still worth noting that a consultant was the first reviewer in only 54% of cases.

Trauma team response

A trauma response was documented in the notes in 69% of ≤16 year olds, slightly higher than the overall data (58%).

Appropriateness of initial response

Table 92 shows advisor assessment of appropriateness of initial hospital response.

Table 92. Appropriateness of initial response depending on patient age

	>16 years		≤16 years	
	Number of patients		Number of patients	
		%		%
Yes	548	86.4	53	88.3
No	86	13.6	7	11.7
Subtotal	**634**		**60**	
Insufficient data	89		8	
Total	**723**		**68**	

Outcome at 72 hours

Six out of 68 paediatric cases (8.8%) were deceased at 72 hours post injury.

Key findings

68/795 (8.6%) cases were aged 16 or less.

Only 54% of cases had consultant staff involved in the immediate management.

The pattern of assessment of overall care was similar to adults with less than half the cases judged as receiving care classified as good practice.

Advanced Paediatric Life Support (APLS) trained staff were not resident or available 24 hours in 20.2% of hospitals.

Only 22 out of 146 hospitals had Registered Sick Children's Nurse cover 24 hours a day, 7 days a week.

Recommendations

All recommendations in this report apply equally to severely injured children.

All sites accepting children for definitive trauma management should have protocols for their management in place. These protocols should be regularly reviewed and updated. *(Hospital trusts)*

All hospitals should have up to date guidelines on the management and referral of suspected non-accidental injury in children. *(Hospital trusts)*

Hospitals should use standard, universal definitions for neonates, infants and children. *(Royal College of Paediatrics and Child Health)*

Each receiving unit should have up to date guidelines for children which recognise the paediatric skills available on site and their limitations and include agreed guidelines for communication and transfer with specialised paediatric services within the local clinical network. *(Strategic health authorities and hospital trusts)*

An Advanced Paediatric Life Support (APLS) (or equivalent) trained consultant and a Registered Sick Children's Nurse (RSCN) or an APLS trained nurse should be involved in the immediate management of all severely injured children. *(Hospital trusts)*

If a hospital does not admit children for definitive care then a bypass protocol should be in place. *(Hospital and ambulance trusts)*

References

1. Services for Children in Emergency departments. Royal College of Paediatrics and Child Health. 2007 *www.rcpch.ac.uk/health-services/emergen-care*

2. The Royal College of Surgeons of England and the British Orthopaedic Society. *Better Care for the Severely Injured.* 2000

CHAPTER 10 - Transfers

Introduction

Most patients with severe injuries are admitted to hospitals that are geographically closest to the location of the incident where the injuries were sustained. Consequently, early management of the patient occurs at centres that may not have the facilities or resources suitable for the appropriate care of the severely injured.

The lack of available appropriate care may result in the transfer to a site with more appropriate facilities. Some ambulance trusts have a policy of bypassing local hospitals to larger trauma centres to obviate the need for later transfer. However, little data supports the fact that such a 'bypass' policy is used with any frequency. In 1997, it was estimated that more than 11,000 patients in the UK with critical illnesses required transfer annually[1].

An example of such a situation is the head injury patient. Approximately 2,200 patients are admitted annually to hospital with head injuries[2]. Of these, 3 – 5% are transferred to regional neurosurgical units for further management. It has been well recognised that the outcome of patients who require a transfer because of a mismatch between the patient's needs and the available resources at the initial place of admission have a better eventual outcome if that transfer is performed by dedicated transport teams[3-6]. However, despite extensive literature highlighting this, in 2002 the Intensive Care Society commented that 'many critically ill patients are transferred between hospitals in an ad hoc manner by inexperienced trainees with little formal supervision and potentially serious complications can occur'[7].

Many studies that have reported on the quality of transfer of patients with head injuries have identified major problems with resuscitation and transfer, including: delays; missed injuries; poor airway management; hypotension; hypoxia; and, the quality of medical escort[8-12].

As a result of these concerns, in 1996, the Association of Anaesthetists of Great Britain and Ireland produced guidelines surrounding the transfer of head injured patients[13]. The main recommendations were:

- **There should be a designated consultant at both the referring and receiving hospitals who have overall responsibility for the transfer of patients.**
- **Local guidelines should be in existence and should be consistent with national guidelines.**
- **Resuscitation and stabilisation of the patient must be achieved before transfer.**
- **Only in exceptional circumstances should a patient with altered conscious level be transferred unintubated.**
- **The doctor accompanying the patient must be of sufficient experience and have received supervised training in the transfer of patients with head injuries.**
- **There must be a means of communication to both the dispatching hospital and the receiving hospital.**

The Intensive Care Society produced guidelines for the transport of the Critically Ill Patient in 1997[14] and then further refined these recommendations in 2002[15]. The recommendations include the following; there should be 'regular meetings of relevant consultants, senior nurses, ambulance providers, bed bureaux managers and commissioners to develop admission and discharge and referral policies and transport protocols, to ensure available resources to enable timely and safe transfers and to develop assurance programmes'.

It was hoped that compliance and subsequent audit of these guidelines, combined with the wider acceptance of the principles and uptake of the Advanced Trauma Life Support (ATLS) approach in the management of patients, would result in an improvement in the quality of transfer. Despite these recommendations, later audits of transfers still revealed inadequacies[11-15].

Results

Only transfers within 72 hours of arrival at hospital were included in the study.

Protocols for secondary transfer

Only 126 of the 183 (68.9%) hospitals involved in the management of patients with severe injuries had protocols for the secondary transfer of patients despite numerous recommendations mandating such protocols.

Number of secondary transfers

Of the 795 patients admitted to hospitals with severe injuries, 194 patients underwent a secondary transfer (24.4%). Eight of these were retrievals with the remaining 186 being transfers conducted by the original admitting hospital.

Effect of mode of initial transport system on secondary transfers

Patients brought to the initial hospital by helicopter were less likely to undergo secondary transfer. Seven out of 59 (11.9%) patients who arrived at the first hospital by helicopter required a secondary transfer within 72 hours of arrival compared with 112/440 (25.5%) patients brought to hospital by road ambulance. The use of helicopters facilitates admission of the severely injured patient to the correct facility initially, thereby reducing subsequent transfers and speeding up definitive care.

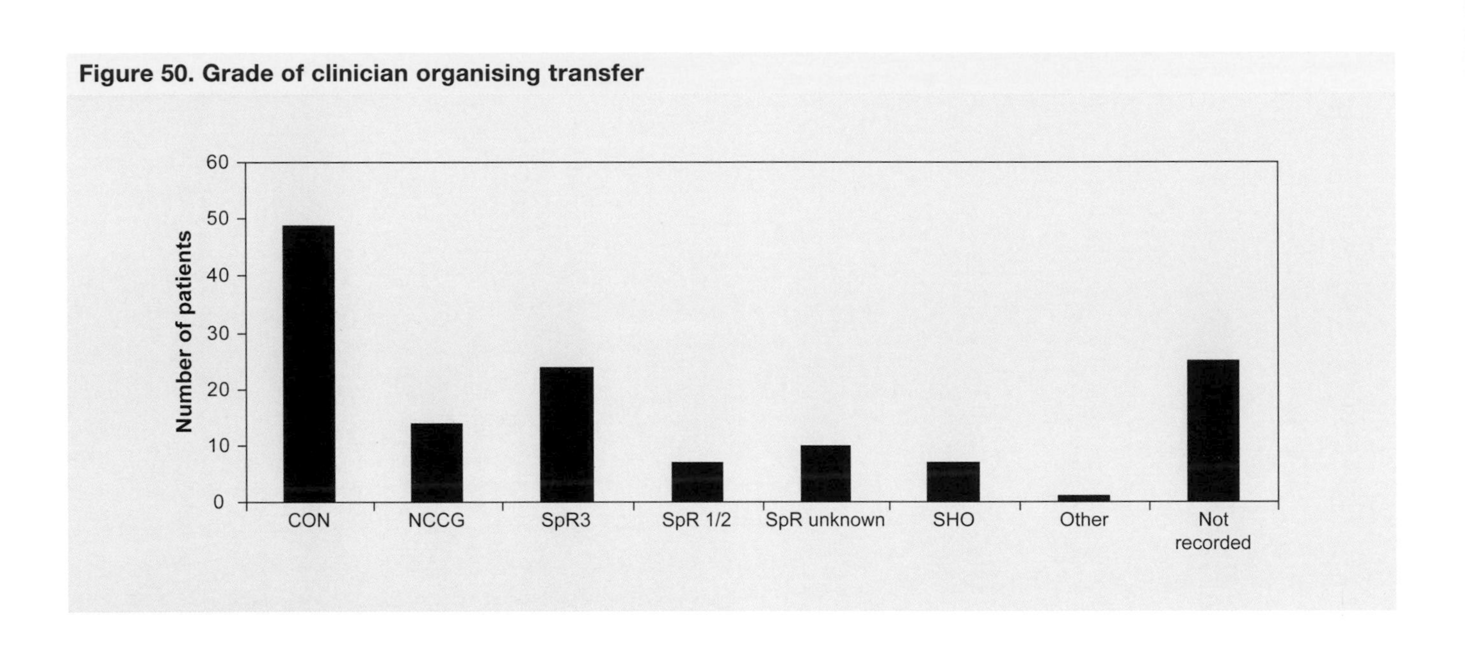

Figure 50. Grade of clinician organising transfer

Table 93. Grade of clinician receiving the transfer

	Number of patients	%
Consultant	14	18.4
NCCG	2	2.6
SpR 3	2	2.6
SpR 1/2	1	1.3
SpR undefined	46	60.5
SHO	10	13.2
Other	1	1.3
Subtotal	**76**	
Not documented	118	
Total	**194**	

Arrangement of transfers

A consultant arranged the transfer in only 49 of 137 (35.8%) cases reported by clinicians on the A&E questionnaire. From the casenotes provided to NCEPOD, the grade of the clinician arranging the transfer could only be identified in 87/194 (44.8%) cases. A consultant was responsible for arranging 39/87 (44.8%) of these transfers (Figure 50).

The documentation of the grade of clinician receiving the patient was equally poorly documented. In 118/194 cases (60.8%) it could not be determined who received the patient. Only 14 cases were documented as being received by consultants (Table 93).

The standards and guidelines for the Transport of the Critically Ill Patient[9] recommends that "each hospital should have a designated consultant available 24 hours a day to organise, supervise and where necessary undertake all inter-hospital transfers" and that the decision to transfer a patient "must be made by a consultant in intensive care in discussion with consultant colleagues". This is not happening. The lack of documented consultant input is a concern. Either local guidelines exist which obviate the need for consultant involvement or the process of care, including transfers, is being managed and delivered by staff in training.

Accompanying staff

Recommendations state that a minimum of two attendants should be present for the transfer[9].

Of the 194 transfers only 35 (18.0%) had a documented second attendant and 3 (1.5%) a third attendant.

In 155/194 cases notified to NCEPOD, the grade of the accompanying person was not documented. In the 39/194 cases where specialty was documented, an anaesthetist or critical care specialist accompanied 36 of the cases. The published recommendations mandate that one of the attendants should be competent in intensive care medicine, anaesthesia or another acute specialty in order to be able to manage any significant airway complication.

Reason for transfer

The reasons for transfer were mainly for specialist management of injuries (172/194; 88.7%). Six patients were transferred due to lack of critical care facilities at the initial hospital. Other reasons cited for transfers were because of lack of local facilities (primarily lack of imaging facilities).

The transfers for specialist care are detailed in Figure 51. Of the 172 cases transferred for specialist treatment, the majority were transferred for neurosurgical care – 106/172 (61.6%). Six (3.5%) patients were transferred to paediatric units. Eighteen (10.5%) patients were transferred for burns/ plastic surgery input and 7 (4.1%) for the management of cardiothoracic injuries.

While it is essential to transfer patients if the appropriate care is not available at the initial receiving hospital, it must be remembered that this will inevitably incur delays in the time to definitive management. In cases where there is a time critical injury e.g. neurosurgical operation for expanding intracranial haematoma, this type of care may not allow

Figure 51. Specialty to which the patients were transferred

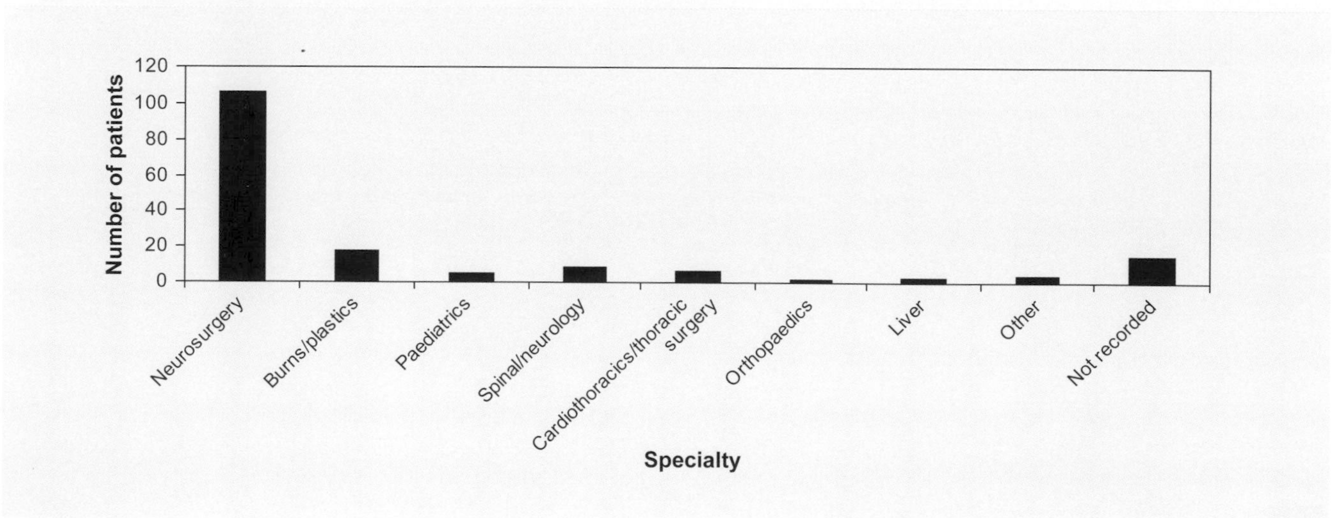

Figure 52. Delay in transfer/retrieval

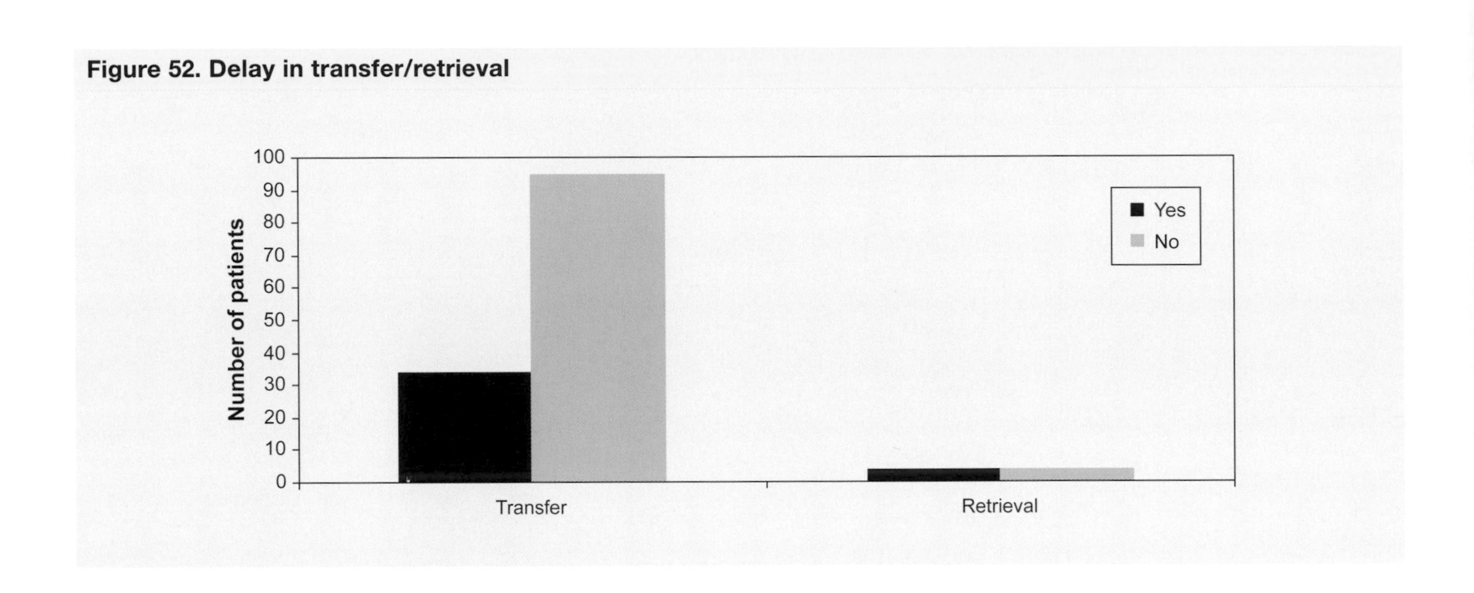

the optimal outcome. Given these clinical considerations and the constraints of staffing in a time of changing training and working hours, it is probably time to consider carefully which hospitals receive severely injured patients and to plan a proper regional trauma service. Patient transport services and the role of doctors in prehospital care must be an integral part of any plans to change trauma services. Both of these plans must occur in parallel as part of a wider trauma care network[12].

Timeliness of transfer

Figure 52 shows information on timeliness of transfer. Where it could be assessed there were delays in 26.4% (34/129) of all transfers and 50% (4/8) of retrievals.

Appropriateness of transfer

Ninety one out of the 194 (46.9%) transfers were considered appropriate by the advisors and 17 (8.8%) transfers were considered inappropriate. There were insufficient or incomplete data to comment and classify the remainder of the transfers.

The reasons identified for the inappropriateness of the transfers included:

transfers with unsurvivable injuries (burns case),

failure of closer centre to accept the patient and, therefore, a longer and delayed transfer was needed,

failures in effective communication between hospitals, and

missed injuries.

Case study 6

A young patient had a severe brain injury following a fall. The patient had a GCS of 3 at presentation with unresponsive pupils and a compound skull fracture with brain matter exuding from the ear. The patient was transferred to a neurosurgical unit but certified brain dead shortly after arrival.

In addition, there were some concerns over the transfer of a number of patients who had sustained a head injury. From the records available six patients with a Glasgow Coma Score of less than 10 were transferred without intubation.

Case study 7

An elderly patient tripped while intoxicated. A Glasgow Coma Score of 3 was recorded in the ambulance. At the receiving hospital it was recoded as 8. The hospital was unable to perform a CT head scan therefore the patient was transferred to the local neurosurgical hospital. The transfer was performed without securing the airway. At the neurosurgical hospital the patient was transferred to CT still with an unprotected airway. Intubation was subsequently performed after CT scanning.

The recommendations on the transfer of patients with head injuries[7] state that only in exceptional circumstances should a patient with a significantly altered conscious level requiring transfer not be sedated, intubated and ventilated.

This review gives a picture of a haphazard arrangement for the secondary transfer of severely injured patients. It is of great concern that one in four patients required secondary transfer to receive definitive care and this must be a major criticism of the current arrangements for the management of severely injured patients. There were deficiencies in local protocols, use of national guidelines, consultant oversight and documentation.

Furthermore, avoidance of transfers by the initial direct transport of the severely injured patient to a centre with the appropriate facilities should be considered. This would need regional planning of all aspects of the trauma service including the prehospital emergency services.

Key findings

There was a lack of adherence to the numerous recommendations and guidelines that exist regarding the transfer of critically ill and severely injured patients.

The arrangements for the secondary transfer of severely injured patients were haphazard.

One in four severely injured patients required a secondary transfer to receive definitive care.

The use of a helicopter system reduced the need for secondary transfers compared to a road ambulance system.

The documentation of transfers was almost uniformly poor.

Despite the limited information available from the poor documentation, there was an apparent lack of consultant input into the arrangement and conduct of secondary transfers.

This study of a three month period suggests that there are approximately 800 transfers annually for severe trauma and that the situation of 'many critically ill patients are transferred between hospitals in an ad hoc manner by inexperienced trainees with little formal supervision and potentially serious complications can occur' is correct. There does not appear to have been any significant change in the last five years.

Recommendations

A clear record of the grade and specialty of all accompanying staff involved in the transfer or retrieval of severely injured patients should be made and this documentation should accompany the patient on transfer. *(Trauma team leader)*

There should be standardised transfer documentation of the patients' details, injuries, results of investigations and management with records kept at the dispatching and receiving hospitals. *(Trauma team leader, Department of Health)*

Published guidelines must be adhered to and audits performed of the transfers and protocols. *(Hospital trusts)*

Local networks should develop protocols for the transfer of severely injured patients suitable for regional requirements. *(Hospital trusts)*

The number of transfers may be decreased if appropriate arrangements are made for cross cover in specialties, e.g. interventional radiology, between trusts. *(Hospital trusts)*

References

1. Mackenzie PA, Smith EA, Wallace PG. *Transfer of adults between intensive care units in the United Kingdom: postal survey.* BMJ. 1997 May 17; 314(7092):1455-6

2 Mendelow et al. *Risks of intracranial haematoma in head Injured Adults.* BMJ 1983; 287:1173

3. McMonagle MP et al. Anz J Surg 2007; 77: 241 – 246

4. Deane SA et al. Anz J Surg 1990; 60: 441-446

5. Strobos J. Ann Emerg Med 1991; 20: 302-310

6. Clemmer TP Crit Care Med 2000; 28: 265-266)

7. Intensive Care Society. Guidelines for transport of the critically ill adult. London: Intensive Care Society 2002

8. Dunn LT. *Secondary insults during the intra hospital transfer of head injured patients: an audit of transfers in the Mersey Region.* Injury 1997; 28:427-31

9. Gentleman D. *Causes and effects of systemic complications among severely head-injured patients transferred to a neurosurgery unit.* Int Surg 1992; 77:297-302

10. Gentleman D et al. *Audit of transfer of unconscious head injured patients to a neurosurgical unit.* Lancet 1990; 335:330-4

11. Have ATLS and national transfer guidelines improved the quality of resuscitation and transfer of head-injured patients? Injury 2003 34:834-838

12. Knowles PR et al. *Meeting the standards for interhospital transfer of adults with severe head injury in the United Kingdom.* Anaesthesia. 1999 Mar; 54(3):283-8

13. AAGBI Recommendations for the transfer of patients with head injuries to neurosurgical injuries. 1996

14. Intensive Care Society. Guidelines for transport of the critically ill adult. London: Intensive care Society 1997

15. Stevenson A et al. *Emergency department organisation of critical care transfers in the UK.* Emerg Med J. 2005 Nov; 22(11):795-8

CHAPTER 11 -
Incidence of trauma and organisation of trauma services

Introduction

Almost all of the evidence of the effectiveness of improvements in the organisation of trauma care services comes from developed countries. In most cases, the better organisation comes in the form of two related activities:

(1) planning of integrated systems for trauma management; and

(2) verification of trauma services through hospital inspections.

Verification applies to a review of individual facilities as regards their provision of a variety of items, including human resources (e.g. availability of personnel with certain qualifications), physical resources (equipment and supplies) and administrative and organisational functions, such as quality improvement, audit (including outcome comparisons) and implementation of protocols (e.g. Advanced Trauma Life Support (ATLS). The American College of Surgeons has made significant progress in this area[1].

The planning of systems for trauma management implies several integrated functions. This includes regional designation of those hospitals able to fulfil the roles of trauma centres at varying levels of complexity; ranging from large urban trauma centres to small rural hospitals and clinics. It also implies the planning of mobile emergency medical services, prehospital triage (to determine which patients should go to which types of designated facilities), transfer criteria and transfer arrangements between hospitals.

Much of the data collected in this study pertains to the first category above (verification). However, the incidence of major trauma in the UK is actually quite low and this has a direct bearing on the ability to provide high quality care to trauma patients. This relationship between volume, quality of care and outcome in trauma has been in the literature for some years[2,3]. This suggests that there is a need to integrate and concentrate major trauma in fewer centres, thus giving a better quality of care.

The incidence of severe trauma defined by an injury severity score of 16 or more is estimated to be four per million per week in the UK[4]; a lower prevalence than in the USA. Burdett-Smith *et al* estimated that there are between 10,000 and 10,600 patients suffering multiple injuries in the UK each year[5]. Given the above estimates, the average acute hospital in the UK is not likely to be called upon to treat more than one severely injured patient each week. Such low numbers suggest that some acute hospitals may have too little experience to give these patients their best chance of optimum outcome. Adequate experience in the definitive management of such difficult problems is hard to acquire without reorganisation of trauma services. Furthermore, it is almost certainly unrealistic to expect every hospital to have the necessary staff and services to be able to provide the standard of care required 24 hours per day, 7 days per week.

Results

In this study, 795 patients with a verified injury severity score of 16 or more were identified over a 12 week period. Table 94 shows data concerning the number of severely injured patients seen by each emergency department in the 12 week study period.

Table 94. Number of patients seen per hospital

	Number of hospitals
1-2	48
3-4	29
5-6	29
7-8	14
9-10	3
11-12	6
13-14	3
15-16	2
17-18	2
19-20	1
> 20	4
Total	**141**

Only 12 emergency departments treated more than one severely injured patient per week during the study period and many departments only treated one to two patients in the whole 12 week study period.

During the study, 243 patients were admitted initially to hospitals that reported 1-5 patients in the study, 226 patients to hospitals that admitted 6-10 patients, 197 patients to hospitals that admitted 11-20 patients to the study and 129 patients to hospitals that admitted more than 20 patients to the study. Figure 53 illustrates the advisors' assessment of overall care analysed by number of patients included in the study.

It can be seen that the high volume hospitals (>20 patients in the study) were assessed as providing a higher percentage of good practice and a lower percentage of all other categories, including insufficient data (Figure 53).

Figure 53. Number of patients per hospital vs. advisors' overall assessment

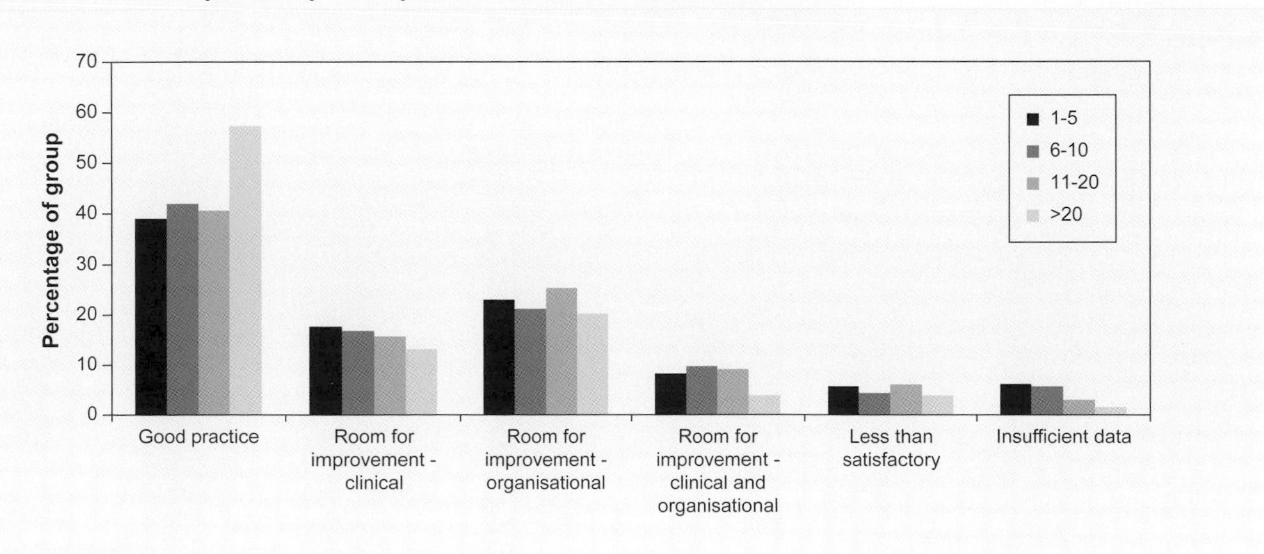

Discussion

The low number of severely injured patients in this study is in keeping with the literature previously referenced. However, these present figures are somewhat lower and this may reflect several factors:

1. Although the study was well publicised and NCEPOD local reporters attempted to collect all cases, it may well be that not all severely injured patients were included in the study.
2. All patients in this study were scored by NCEPOD staff, and patients who were identified as severely injured by the participating centre but who subsequently had an injury severity score (ISS) <16 were excluded from the study.
3. The incidence of severe trauma appears to be falling in England and Wales, presumably due to education or public health measures and factors such as better vehicle and road design.

Despite recent improvements, it appears that the outcome from severe trauma in the UK remains poorer than in other developed countries. Furthermore, it appears that the improvements in mortality for severely injured patients occurred between 1989 and 1994 and that no significant change occurred between 1994 and 2000[6]. This study also showed that consultant involvement increased from 29% to 40% over 1989-1994 but did not increase further up to the year 2000.

It may be that the benefits of an Advanced Trauma Life Support (ATLS) approach have delivered maximum improvements for the severely injured patient within the current system of trauma care and that further improvements in outcome for patients who have suffered major trauma cannot be delivered by focusing only on improving the quality of care within current institutions but must also take into account the regional organisation of trauma services. A number of reports have suggested regionalisation of trauma care[7-10] over the last two decades but with little impact on service provision. **Changing the provision of trauma services is urgently required[11].**

This report has highlighted major deficiencies in the management of the severely injured patient. Many of these deficiencies were organisational and should not be taken as a comment on the ability or willingness of individual clinicians to provide a high standard of care.

These data have highlighted deficiencies or problems in the following areas:

Trauma team and trauma response (page 51-55)

One in five hospitals did not have a trauma team.

Only three out of five severely injured patients are met by a trauma team.

Consultant involvement (page 55-58)

A consultant was the trauma team leader/first reviewer in only one in four cases.

Consultants were involved in the initial care of four out of 10 patients presenting during daytime but only one out of 10 patients presenting at night.

One in three patients were not seen by a consultant whilst in the emergency department.

Neurosurgery (page 102-107)

One hundred and fourteen patients required neurosurgery as a result of head trauma. Fifty eight of these patients (50.9%) were initially taken to a non-neurosurgical centre. Only one out of seven of these patients had surgery within four hours. Two out of three patients taken initially to a neurosurgical centre had surgery within four hours of injury.

Availability of interventional radiology (page 25-33 and page 98-102)

The use of interventional radiology has an increasing role in the management of haemorrhage in the trauma patient. Only one patient in this study underwent an interventional radiology technique. Only six out of 10 hospitals stated that they had 24 hour access to this therapy and in many of those this is ad hoc due to the small number of trained individuals.

Secondary transfers (page 118-124)

One in four severely injured patients required a secondary transfer to receive definitive care. This underlines the inability of the original admitting facility to provide definitive care. Furthermore, these transfers were conducted in a haphazard fashion with little consultant oversight.

Prehospital airway management (page 37-48)

One in 10 patients arrived at hospital with an obstructed or partially obstructed airway.

Eleven out of 85 attempted prehospital intubations failed (12.9%). Eight of these patients were dead at 72 hours post injury (72.7% mortality rate).

These six issues have been used for illustrative purposes only. It can be appreciated that not every hospital can have the manpower, facilities, equipment and expertise to provide definitive care for all severely injured patients. Furthermore, many of the problems that exist in trauma management, including the prehospital phase, are organisational and do not reflect on the abilities or enthusiasm of clinical teams. The infrequent incidence of major trauma compounds these issues.

As previously referenced, and shown in this study (Figure 53), there is an association between the volume of cases and good outcomes[2,3]. It is also known that patients who are admitted directly to a trauma centre have less morbidity and a lower mortality than patients who are initially admitted to a more local hospital and subsequently transferred to a trauma centre[12].

Regional reconfiguration of trauma services will allow the concentration of relatively few patients in limited number of centres that could develop their expertise. This will ensure that all the staff, facilities, equipment and expertise to manage these challenging patients will be immediately available. Sustainable rotas will be deliverable and will ensure better availability of consultants and other staff at all times. There will be more efficient use of limited resources and it appears that the societal cost of such a system is favourable [13]. Concentration of major trauma will give opportunities to increase the robustness of audit and quality control and will also facilitate much needed research in this area. The current draft of National Institute for Health and Clinical Excellence (NICE) guidance on head injury management included a research question about the benefit of direct transfer of head injured patients to neurosurgical centres.

However, the current system is likely to change slowly. Even in a system of more regionalised trauma care there will be many patients presenting to and managed at a number of different hospitals within a region. All hospitals within a region have a major part to play in the management of the injured patient.

Under the current system where there is little regionalisation, the role of the district general hospital is crucial. All hospitals have a major role in the initial management, stabilisation, and identification of injuries and provision of definitive care where possible. Too often the district general hospitals perceive their role to be solely the organisation of secondary transfer to an 'ivory tower'. This can result in the focus of care being the transfer rather than the immediate management of the unstable patient.

Trauma audit

The care of the severely injured patient requires a multidisciplinary team, often working across more than one hospital. This is different from most other types of medical care (where usually only one specialist is involved) and means that special arrangements have to be made to develop a system that coordinates the complex interactions between the different individuals involved in trauma care. To show whether or not these arrangements are working well, a robust audit system is required – ideally evaluating both processes and outcomes. A key part of a trauma system is the multidisciplinary trauma audit meeting, where all those involved in trauma care can meet to discuss both individual patient management and the overall performance of the trauma system. This type of audit is more effective if the data presented for discussion allows comparisons with other hospitals (benchmarking) to occur.

Trauma audit follows this benchmarking pattern in America, Germany, Scandinavia and Australia. In the USA, trauma outcome audit has become a mandatory requirement for trauma centre status. In the UK, the Trauma Audit and Research Network (TARN) is a well-established process and outcome audit in trauma care, which was originally derived from the methods used in the American Major Trauma Outcome Study (MTOS). TARN data is used in three ways to close the cycle of trauma audit:

1) To highlight individual cases where unexpected outcomes occur (either good or bad). This allows multidisciplinary trauma audit meetings to focus on the particular cases that are most likely to contain the lessons for improvement.

2) Four times a year the Quarterly Report focuses on a particular specialist area of trauma management – comparing performance with standards set by the Royal College of Surgeons Trauma Committee and also benchmarking performance of one hospital against the rest of the UK. This information usually forms the basis for a departmental or multidisciplinary trauma audit meeting.

3) Comparisons of outcome between hospitals can be made, and are publicly available to purchasers and service users through the Healthcare Commission website, along with case mix data by hospital. This allows the identification of 'outliers' with either very good or very poor trauma outcomes, allowing potential causes to be identified.

TARN is a voluntary system, funded by subscription from participating hospitals. It has data from about 50% of UK hospitals; with about one third participating at any one time.

The database collected by TARN now contains about 200,000 patient records, so it can also be used for various types of research and to look at long-term trends in trauma outcomes[14-17].

In this study, 183 hospitals returned an organisational questionnaire. Of these 183 hospitals, only 77 (42.1%) participated in, and provided data to, TARN.

Key findings

129/141 (91.5%) hospitals in this study dealt with a severely injured patient less often than once per week.

High volume hospitals (>20 severely injured patients in this study) deliver a higher percentage of care assessed as good practice.

Only 77/183 (42.1%) hospitals participate in TARN.

Recommendations

A system should be initiated for identifying these patients so that the demand on the health service can be properly quantified and resources appropriate to that demand be made available. *(Department of Health)*

Given the relatively low incidence of severe trauma in the UK, it is unlikely that each individual hospital can deliver optimum care to this challenging group of patients. Regional planning for the effective delivery of trauma services is therefore essential. *(Strategic health authorities, hospital trusts)*

Given the importance of evaluation of processes and outcomes in the trauma patient, all units providing treatment for severely injured patients should contribute to the Trauma Audit Research Network. *(Hospital trusts)*

There should be a system of designation and verification of each hospital with regards to their function as a trauma centre, in a similar fashion to the system instituted by the American College of Surgeons. *(Strategic health authorities, Royal College of Surgeons)*

References

1. *www.facs.org/trauma/verificationhosp.html*

2. Nathens AB, Jurkovich GJ, Maler RV et al. *Relationship between trauma centre volume and outcomes.* JAMA 2001; 285: 1164-71

3. MacKenzie EJ et al. *A national evaluation of the effect of trauma centre care on mortality* NEJM 2006; 354: 366-378

4. Gorman et al. *The epidemiology of major injuries in Mersey and North Wales.* Injury. 1995 26; 1 51-54

5. Burdett-Smith P, Airey GM, and Franks AJ. *Improvement in trauma survival in Leeds.* Injury. 1995 26; 7.455-458.

6. Lecky FE, Woodford M, Bouamra O, Yates DW. *Lack of change in trauma care in England and Wales since 1994.* Emerg Med J. 2002 Nov; 19(6):520-3

7. Commission on the Provision of Surgical Services. *The Management of Patients with Major Injuries.* The Royal College of Surgeons of England; 1988

8. The Management of Skeletal Trauma in the United Kingdom. British Orthopaedic Association. London; 1992

9. The Care of Severely Injured Patients in the United Kingdom. British Orthopaedic Association. London; 1997

10. The Royal College of Surgeons of England and the British Orthopaedic Society. Better Care for the Severely Injured. 2000

11. *http://www.healthcareforlondon.nhs.uk/framework_for_action.asp*

12. Sampalis JS, Denis R, Fréchette P, Brown R, Fleiszer D, Mulder D. *Direct transport to tertiary trauma centers versus transfer from lower level facilities: impact on mortality and morbidity among patients with major trauma.* J Trauma. 1997 Aug; 43(2):288-95

13. Durham R, Pracht E, Orban B, Lottenburg L, Tepas J, Flint L. *Evaluation of a mature trauma system.* Ann Surg. 2006; 243(6):775-83

14. Lecky FE, Woodford M, Bouamra O, Yates DW. *Lack of change in trauma care in England and Wales since 1994.* Emergency Medical Journal 2002; 19:0-3

15. Patel HC, Woodford M, King AT, Yates DW, Lecky FE. *Trends in head injury outcome from 1989 to 2003 and the effect of neurosurgical care: an observational study on behalf of the Trauma Audit & Research Network.* The Lancet 2005; 366: 1538-44

16. Dark P, Woodford M, Vail A, Mackway-Jones K, Yates D, Lecky F. *Systolic hypertension and the response to blunt trauma in infants and children.* Resuscitation 2002; 54: 245-253

17. Henderson K, Coats TJ, Hassan TB, Brohi K. *Audit of time to emergency trauma laparotomy.* Br J Surg 2000; 87: 472-476

APPENDIX A - Glossary

A&E	Accident and Emergency
ABC	Airway, breathing, circulation
ABG	Arterial blood gas
APLS	Advanced paediatric life support
ATLS	Advanced trauma life support
AVPU	Alert, verbal, pain, unresponsive
CT	Computed tomography
DPL	Diagnostic peritoneal lavage
FAST	Focussed Assessment with Sonography for Trauma
GCS	Glasgow coma score / scale
ICP	Intracranial pressure
ICU	Intensive care unit
ISS	Injury severity score
IV	Intra venous
JRCALC	Joint Royal Colleges Ambulance Liaison Committee
kPa	Kilo Pascals
mmHg	Millimetres of Mercury
MTOS	Major Trauma Outcome Study
NCCG	Non consultant career grade
NHS	National Health Service
NICE	National Institute for Health and Clinical Excellence
OPCS	Office of Population, Censuses and Surveys
$PaCO_2$	Partial pressure of Carbon Dioxide
PaO_2	Partial pressure of Oxygen
PRF	Patient report form
RCS	Royal College of Surgeons of England
RSCN	Registered sick children's nurse
RTC	Road traffic collision
SHO	Senior house officer
SIGN	Scottish Intercollegiate Guidelines Network
$SpCO_2$	Saturation of peripheral Carbon Dioxide
SpO_2	Saturation of peripheral Oxygen
SpR	Specialist registrar
TARN	Trauma Audit Research Network

APPENDIX B - Injury severity score

Abbreviated Injury Scale

The Abbreviated Injury Scale (AIS) is an anatomical scoring system first introduced in 1969. Injuries are ranked on a scale of 1 to 6, with 1 being minor, 5 severe and 6 an unsurvivable injury. This represents the 'threat to life' associated with an injury and is not meant to represent a comprehensive measure of severity. The AIS is not an injury scale, in that the difference between AIS1 and AIS2 is not the same as that between AIS4 and AIS5.

AIS Score	Injury
1	Minor
2	Moderate
3	Serious
4	Severe
5	Critical
6	Unsurvivable

Injury Severity Score

The Injury Severity Score (ISS) is an anatomical scoring system that provides an overall score for patients with multiple injuries. Each injury is assigned an **Abbreviated Injury Scale** (AIS) score and is allocated to one of six body regions (Head, Face, Chest, Abdomen, Extremities (including Pelvis), External). Only the highest AIS score in each body region is used. The three most severely injured body regions have their score squared and added together to produce the ISS score.

An example of the ISS calculation is shown below:

Region	Injury Description	AIS	Square Top Three
Head & Neck	Cerebral Contusion	3	9
Face	No Injury	0	
Chest	Flail Chest	4	16
Abdomen	Minor Contusion of Liver Complex Rupture Spleen	2 5	25
Extremity	Fractured femur	3	
External	No Injury	0	
	Injury Severity Score:		**50**

The ISS score takes values from 0 to 75. If an injury is assigned an AIS of 6 (unsurvivable injury), the ISS score is automatically assigned to 75. The ISS score correlates linearly with mortality, morbidity, hospital stay and other measures of severity.

Tables and information taken from *http://www.trauma.org/scores/ais.html* and *http://www.trauma.org/scores/iss.html*

APPENDIX C - Adult and paediatric Glasgow Coma Scale

The Glasgow Coma Scale and Coma Score (GCS)

For clarity the Glasgow Coma Scale and Glasgow Coma Score are described below.

The Glasgow Coma Scale provides a framework for describing the state of a patient in terms of three aspects of responsiveness: eye opening, verbal response, and best motor response, each stratified according to increasing impairment. In the first description of the Scale for general use, the motor response had only five options, with no demarcation between 'normal' and 'abnormal' flexion. The distinction between these movements can be difficult to make consistently and is rarely useful in monitoring an individual patient but is relevant to prognosis and is, therefore, part of an extended six option scale used to classify severity in groups of patients.

The Glasgow Coma Score is an artificial index; obtained by adding scores for the three responses. The notation for the score was derived from the extended scale, incorporating the distinction between normal and abnormal flexion movements, producing a total score of 15. This score can provide a useful single figure summary and a basis for systems of classification, but contains less information than a description separately of the three responses.

The three responses of the coma scale, not the total score, should therefore be of use in describing, monitoring and exchanging information about individual patients.

Table Glasgow Coma Scale and Score (Adults)

Feature	Scale responses	Score notation
Eye opening	Spontaneous	4
	To speech	3
	To pain	2
	None	1
Verbal response	Orientated	5
	Confused conversation	4
	Words (inappropriate)	3
	Sounds (incomprehensible)	2
	None	1
Best motor response	Obey commands	6
	Localise pain	5
	Flexion - Normal	4
	- Abnormal	3
	Extend	2
	None	1
	Total coma score	**3/15 - 15/15**

Paediatric Glasgow Coma Scale

The paediatric version of the Glasgow Coma Scale is modified from the Adult Glasgow Coma Scale to take into account of problems assessing the Best Verbal Response in pre-verbal patients.

It is composed of three parameters: Best Eye Response, Best Verbal Response and Best Motor Response. The definition of these parameters is given below.

Best Eye Response (4)

4. Eyes open spontaneously
3. Eye opening to verbal command
2. Eye opening to pain
1. No eye opening

Best Verbal Response (5)

5. Alert, babbles, coos, words or sentences to usual ability
4. Less than usual ability and/or spontaneous irritable cry
3. Cries inappropriately
2. Occasionally whimpers and/or moans
1. No vocal response

Communication with the infant or child's caregivers is required to establish the best usual verbal response. A 'grimace' alternative to verbal responses should be used in pre-verbal or intubated patients.

Best Grimace Response (5)

5. Spontaneous normal facial/oro-motor activity
4. Less than usual spontaneous ability or only response to touch stimuli
3. Vigorous grimace to pain
2. Mild grimace to pain
1. No response to pain

Best Motor Response (6)

6. Obeys commands or performs normal spontaneous movements
5. Localises to painful stimuli or withdraws to touch
4. Withdrawal to painful stimuli
3. Abnormal flexion to pain
2. Abnormal extension to pain
1. No motor response to pain

Classification of severity of head injury using GCS

Whilst the individual components of the Glasgow Coma Scale should be used in communication about individual patients the use of the aggregate Glasgow Coma Score can be useful for describing patient populations.

The use of the aggregate score does allow the severity of head injury to be classified into the following categories:

Minor	GCS	15
Mild	GCS	13-14
Moderate	GCS	9-12
Severe	GCS	3-8

These classifications allow easy description of a head injured population and are used within this text.

For some data presentation patients with GCS equal to 3 have been separated out from the rest of the severe head injury group (GCS 4-8). This has been done to help understand that data more easily as it is know that patients with GCS equal to 3 have a much poorer prognosis than the rest of the severe head injured group.

APPENDIX D - An example of an excellent Patient Report Form (PRF)

Incident Number

Date D D / M M / Y Y

Attendant PIN

Driver

Callsign

Activated From

Base

H H M M

Mobile :

At scene :

Left scene :

At hospital :

Clear :

Name and Address

Postcode M F

D D M M Y Y Age

DOB / /

Contact details

GP's Name

Incident type

999

Drs call

Other

Chief complaint

Location

History of incident

Time of onset /incident :

MPDS Codes Given

Actual

Work

Home

Leisure

Also at scene:

Fire Doctor

Police Other

Allergies None Unknown

Medications None Unknown

Past Medical History None Unknown

H H M M

Last meal (Time) :

Events (leading to onset) None Unknown

Details of AMPLE

RTA

Pedestrian

Cyclist

Motorcyclist

Vehicle occupant (mark location)

	Y	N
Helmet worn		
Seatbelt worn		
Child restraint		
Head restraint		
Airbag opened		
Ejected		
Fatality in same vehicle		
Trapped		

Duration

H H M M

:

Primary Survey

Airway

Clear Obstruction

Aspirated

C-Spine

Normal Suspect

Breathing

Present Absent

Normal Abnormal

Pulse

Present Absent

Regular Irregular

Strong Weak

Capillary refill

Normal >2sec

AVPU

Alert Voice

Pain

Unresponsive

Examination

Mark injury on diagram

C losed #

O pen #

P ain

L aceration

F oreign body

A brasion

E chymoses

B urns

% Area burns

Pulse distal to limb injury? Y N

Skin

Normal

Cyanosed

Pale

Flushed

Sweating

Breath sounds

	Right	Left
Normal		
Abnormal		
Reduced		
Absent		

	Y	N
Nausea		
Vomiting		
Fitting		
KO'd?		
Alcohol?		

Mark damage **X X X** / Mark direction of impact →

This is to certify that, despite Ambulance advice I have declined;

Treatment To attend hospital To wear a seatbelt

I hereby absolve the Ambulance Service from any responsibility that may arise from my refusal.

Refused to sign

Signed

Obs. /Times	H H : M M	H H : M M	H H : M M
Pulse			
BP systolic			
diastolic			
Resp Rate			
SpO2%			
Peak flow			
BM	.	.	.
Pupils	R L	R L	R L
Reaction (Y/N)			
Size (N/C/D)			

GCS /Times HH : MM | HH : MM | HH : MM

Form No. 96514

Eye Opening
- Spontaneous 4
- To voice 3
- To pain 2
- None 1

VERBAL
- Orientated 5
- Confused 4
- Inappropriate 3
- Incomprehensible 2
- None 1

MOTOR (Right / Left)
- Obeys 6
- Localises 5
- Withdraws 4
- Flexion 3
- Extension 2
- None 1

Total

Cardiac Monitor ☐ ☐ 12 Lead ECG **(Attach strip)**

Rhythm(s)
NSR ☐ Brady ☐ Tachy ☐ Other ☐
VT ☐ VF ☐ Asystole ☐ PEA ☐

Cardiac Arrest ☐
Witnessed? CPR Time of arrest HH : MM
By bystander ☐ ☐
By Amb Crew ☐ ☐ MCCU Summoned ☐
Defibrillation ☐ Initial rhythm VF ☐ ☐ VT
No. shocks X Energy J By
No. shocks X Energy J By

Rhythm Outcome
NSR ☐ VF ☐ Brady ☐ PEA ☐
Tachy ☐ Asystole ☐ VT ☐ other ☐
Defibrillation successful (return of spontaneous circulation) ☐

Management
- Headtilt/chin lift
- Jaw thrust
- Manual clearance
- Suction
- Nasal Airway
- OP Airway
- Pocket mask
- Bag & Mask
- Ventilator
- Entonox
- C- collar
- Control bleeding
- Cricothyroidotomy
- Chest decompression
- Intraosseous needle
- Spinal board
- RED
- Orthopaedic stretcher
- Vacuum Mattress
- Rescue strecher
- Vacuum splint
- Box splint
- Traction splint
- Other splinting
- Frac straps

Intubation ☐
Unsuccessful ☐
Size .
By

Cannulation ☐
Unsuccessful ☐
Size G
2nd G
By

Management Comments

Oxygen therapy ☐

Drug/ Fluid **/Route** IV ET SC IM Other
- Epinephrine 1:10.000
- Lidocaine
- Atropine 3mg
- Atropine 500mcg
- IV Saline flush 2ml
- IV Saline 500ml
- IV Gelofusine 500ml
- Nalbuphine (Nubain)
- Naloxone (Narcan)
- Glucagon
- Epinephrine 1:1,000
- Diazepam 10mg PR
- Diazepam 5mg PR
- Salbutamol 2.5mg Neb.
- Salbutamol 5mg Neb.
- GTN - Suscard Buccal 2mg Buccal
- Aspirin 300mg Oral
- Other(s) - Name & Dose Route

	Drug & dose	Time of admin.	By
1		:	
2		:	
3		:	
4		:	
5		:	
6		:	
7		:	
8		:	
9		:	
10		:	

Transported to: Hospital ☐
A&E ☐ CCU ☐ Other dept. ☐
DOA ☐ Left at scene ☐

Signed

APPENDIX E - Level 1 trauma care

As defined in Better Care for the Severely Injured. A Report from the Royal College of Surgeons of England and the British Orthopaedic Society. 2000

The Required Facilities at the Major Acute Hospitals (Level 1)

A 24-hour resuscitative trauma team, led by a consultant with current ATLS® certification or equivalent, must be in place.

A 24-hour, fully staffed A&E department, supported by on-call A&E consultants, supported by specialist registrars.

ICU beds and trauma beds on the same site as the A&E department.

On-site 24-hour X-ray and CT scanning with appropriate staffing and immediate reporting facilities.

The equivalent of four to eight whole-time consultants exclusively dealing with orthopaedic trauma.

A dedicated trauma theatre and daily consultant orthopaedic trauma lists.

A helicopter pad close to the A&E department is mandatory. There should be no additional secondary journey by road. The helicopter landing site should allow landing throughout the 24 hours.

There must be on-site departments of:

- **Orthopaedic trauma**
- **Neurosurgery**
- **General and vascular surgery**
- **Plastic surgery**
- **Cardiothoracic or thoracic surgery**
- **Head & neck surgery**
- **Urology**
- **Anaesthesia with intensive care**
- **Interventional radiology**
- **Paediatric surgery**
- **Intensive care beds for children**
- **A named consultant director of trauma.**

APPENDIX F - Participation

Trust	Cases identified	Organisational questionnaire returned
Aintree Hospitals NHS Trust	Yes	Yes
Airedale NHS Trust	Yes	Yes
Ashford & St Peter's Hospital NHS Trust	Yes	Yes
Barking, Havering and Redbridge Hospitals NHS Trust	Yes	Yes
Barnet and Chase Farm Hospitals NHS Trust	No	Yes
Barnsley Hospital NHS Foundation Trust	Yes	Yes
Barts and The London NHS Trust	Yes	Yes
Basildon & Thurrock University Hospitals NHS FoundationTrust	Yes	Yes
Basingstoke & North Hampshire Hospitals NHS Foundation Trust	Yes	Yes
Bedford Hospital NHS Trust	Yes	Yes
Birmingham Childrens Hospital NHS Trust	Yes	Yes
Blackpool, Fylde and Wyre Hospitals NHS Trust	Yes	Yes
Bolton Hospitals NHS Trust	Yes	Yes
Bradford Teaching Hospitals NHS Foundation Trust	Yes	Yes
Brighton and Sussex University Hospitals NHS Trust	Yes	Yes
Bro Morgannwg NHS Trust	Yes	Yes
Bromley Hospitals NHS Trust	Yes	Yes
Buckinghamshire Hospitals NHS Trust	No	Yes
Burton Hospitals NHS Trust	Yes	Yes
Calderdale & Huddersfield NHS Trust	Yes	No
Cambridge University Hospitals NHS Foundation Trust	Yes	Yes
Cardiff and Vale NHS Trust	Yes	Yes
Carmarthenshire NHS Trust	Yes	Yes
Central Manchester/Manchester Childrens Univ Hosps NHST	Yes	Yes
Ceredigion & Mid Wales NHS Trust	Yes	Yes
Chelsea & Westminster Healthcare NHS Trust	Yes	No

APPENDIX F - Participation

Trust	Cases identified	Organisational questionnaire returned
Chesterfield Royal Hospital NHS Foundation Trust	Yes	Yes
City Hospitals Sunderland NHS Foundation Trust	Yes	Yes
Conwy & Denbighshire NHS Trust	Yes	Yes
Countess of Chester Hospital NHS Foundation Trust	Yes	Yes
County Durham and Darlington Acute Hospitals NHS Trust	Yes	Yes
Craigavon Area Hospital Group Trust	Yes	Yes
Dartford & Gravesham NHS Trust	Yes	Yes
Derby Hospitals NHS Foundation Trust	Yes	Yes
Doncaster and Bassetlaw Hospitals NHS Foundation Trust	Yes	Yes
Dorset County Hospital NHS Foundation Trust	Yes	Yes
Down Lisburn Health & Social Services Trust	No	Yes
Dudley Group of Hospitals NHS Trust	Yes	Yes
Ealing Hospital NHS Trust	Yes	Yes
East & North Hertfordshire NHS Trust	Yes	Yes
East Cheshire NHS Trust	Yes	Yes
East Kent Hospitals NHS Trust	Yes	Yes
East Lancashire Hospitals NHS Trust	No	No
East Sussex Hospitals NHS Trust	Yes	Yes
Epsom and St Helier University Hospitals NHS Trust	Yes	Yes
Essex Rivers Healthcare NHS Trust	Yes	Yes
Frimley Park Hospitals NHS Trust	Yes	Yes
Gateshead Health NHS Trust	No	Yes
George Eliot Hospital NHS Trust	Yes	Yes
Gloucestershire Hospitals NHS Foundation Trust	Yes	Yes
Good Hope Hospital NHS Trust	Yes	No
Guy's & St Thomas' NHS Foundation Trust	Yes	Yes

Trust	Cases identified	Organisational questionnaire returned
Gwent Healthcare NHS Trust	Yes	Yes
Hammersmith Hospitals NHS Trust	Yes	Yes
Harrogate and District NHS Foundation Trust	Yes	Yes
Health & Social Services, States of Guernsey	Yes	Yes
Heart of England NHS Foundation Trust	Yes	Yes
Heatherwood and Wexham Park Hospitals NHS Trust	Yes	Yes
Hereford Hospitals NHS Trust	Yes	Yes
Hillingdon Hospital NHS Trust	No	Yes
Hinchingbrooke Health Care NHS Trust	No	Yes
Homerton University Hospital NHS Foundation Trust	Yes	Yes
Hull and East Yorkshire Hospitals NHS Trust	Yes	Yes
Ipswich Hospital NHS Trust	No	Yes
Isle of Man Department of Health & Social Security	Yes	Yes
Isle of Wight Healthcare NHS Trust	Yes	Yes
James Paget Healthcare NHS Trust	Yes	Yes
Kettering General Hospital NHS Trust	Yes	Yes
King's College Hospital NHS Trust	Yes	Yes
Kingston Hospital NHS Trust	Yes	Yes
Lancashire Teaching Hospitals NHS Foundation Trust	No	No
Leeds Teaching Hospitals NHS Trust (The)	Yes	Yes
Lewisham Hospital NHS Trust	Yes	Yes
Luton and Dunstable Hospital NHS Trust	No	Yes
Maidstone and Tunbridge Wells NHS Trust	Yes	Yes
Mater Hospital Belfast Health & Social Services Trust	Yes	Yes
Mayday Health Care NHS Trust	Yes	Yes
Medway NHS Trust	No	Yes

APPENDIX F - Participation

Trust	Cases identified	Organisational questionnaire returned
Mid Cheshire Hospitals NHS Trust	Yes	Yes
Mid Staffordshire General Hospitals NHS Trust	Yes	Yes
Mid Yorkshire Hospitals NHS Trust	Yes	Yes
Mid-Essex Hospital Services NHS Trust	No	Yes
Milton Keynes General NHS Trust	Yes	Yes
Newcastle upon Tyne Hospitals NHS Foundation Trust	Yes	Yes
Newham Healthcare NHS Trust	Yes	No
Norfolk & Norwich University Hospital NHS Trust	Yes	Yes
North Bristol NHS Trust	Yes	Yes
North Cheshire Hospitals NHS Trust	Yes	Yes
North Cumbria Acute Hospitals NHS Trust	Yes	No
North East Wales NHS Trust	No	Yes
North Glamorgan NHS Trust	No	No
North Middlesex University Hospital NHS Trust	Yes	Yes
North Tees and Hartlepool NHS Trust	Yes	Yes
North West London Hospitals NHS Trust	Yes	Yes
North West Wales NHS Trust	No	Yes
Northampton General Hospital NHS Trust	Yes	Yes
Northern Devon Healthcare NHS Trust	Yes	Yes
Northern Lincolnshire & Goole Hospitals Trust	Yes	Yes
Northumbria Healthcare NHS Trust	Yes	Yes
Nottingham University Hospitals NHS Trust	Yes	Yes
Oxford Radcliffe Hospital NHS Trust	Yes	Yes
Pembrokeshire & Derwen NHS Trust	Yes	Yes
Pennine Acute Hospitals NHS Trust (The)	Yes	Yes
Peterborough & Stamford Hospitals NHS Foundation Trust	Yes	Yes

Trust	Cases identified	Organisational questionnaire returned
Plymouth Hospitals NHS Trust	Yes	Yes
Pontypridd & Rhondda NHS Trust	No	Yes
Poole Hospital NHS Trust	No	No
Portsmouth Hospitals NHS Trust	Yes	Yes
Princess Alexandra Hospital NHS Trust	No	No
Queen Elizabeth Hospital NHS Trust	Yes	Yes
Queen Mary's Sidcup NHS Trust	Yes	Yes
Royal Berkshire NHS Foundation Trust	Yes	Yes
Royal Bournemouth and Christchurch Hospitals NHS Trust	Yes	Yes
Royal Cornwall Hospitals NHS Trust	Yes	Yes
Royal Devon and Exeter NHS Foundation Trust	Yes	Yes
Royal Free Hampstead NHS Trust	Yes	Yes
Royal Group of Hospitals & Dental Hospitals & Maternity Hosp	Yes	Yes
Royal Liverpool & Broadgreen University Hospitals NHS Trust	Yes	Yes
Royal Liverpool Children's NHS Trust	Yes	Yes
Royal Surrey County Hospital NHS Trust	Yes	Yes
Royal United Hospital Bath NHS Trust	Yes	Yes
Royal West Sussex NHS Trust	Yes	No
Royal Wolverhampton Hospitals NHS Trust (The)	Yes	Yes
Salford Royal Hospitals NHS Trust	Yes	Yes
Salisbury Foundation NHS Trust	Yes	Yes
Sandwell and West Birmingham Hospitals NHS Trust	Yes	Yes
Scarborough and North East Yorkshire Health Care NHS Trust	Yes	Yes
Sheffield Children's NHS Foundation Trust	Yes	No
Sheffield Teaching Hospitals NHS Foundation Trust	Yes	Yes
Sherwood Forest Hospitals NHS Trust	Yes	No

APPENDIX F - Participation

Trust	Cases identified	Organisational questionnaire returned
Shrewsbury and Telford Hospitals NHS Trust	Yes	Yes
South Devon Healthcare NHS Trust	Yes	Yes
South Tees Hospitals NHS Trust	Yes	Yes
South Tyneside NHS Foundation Trust	Yes	Yes
South Warwickshire General Hospitals NHS Trust	No	No
Southampton University Hospitals NHS Trust	Yes	Yes
Southend Hospital NHS Trust	Yes	Yes
Southport and Ormskirk Hospitals NHS Trust	Yes	Yes
Sperrin Lakeland Health & Social Care NHS Trust	No	Yes
St George's Healthcare NHS Trust	Yes	Yes
St Helens and Knowsley Hospitals NHS Trust	Yes	Yes
St Mary's NHS Trust	Yes	Yes
States of Jersey Health & Social Services	Yes	Yes
Stockport NHS Foundation Trust	Yes	Yes
Surrey & Sussex Healthcare NHS Trust	Yes	Yes
Swansea NHS Trust	Yes	Yes
Swindon & Marlborough NHS Trust	Yes	Yes
Tameside and Glossop Acute Services NHS Trust	Yes	Yes
Taunton & Somerset NHS Trust	Yes	Yes
The Queen Elizabeth Hospital King's Lynn NHS Trust	Yes	Yes
The Rotherham NHS Foundation Trust	Yes	Yes
Trafford Healthcare NHS Trust	Yes	Yes
Ulster Community & Hospitals NHS Trust	No	Yes
United Bristol Healthcare NHS Trust	Yes	Yes
United Hospitals Health & Social Services Trust	Yes	Yes
United Lincolnshire Hospitals NHS Trust	Yes	Yes

Trust	Cases identified	Organisational questionnaire returned
Univ. Hospital of South Manchester NHS Foundation Trust	Yes	Yes
University College London Hospitals NHS Foundation Trust	No	Yes
University Hospital Birmingham NHS Foundation Trust	Yes	Yes
University Hospital of North Staffordshire NHS Trust	No	No
University Hospitals Coventry and Warwickshire NHS Trust	Yes	Yes
University Hospitals of Leicester NHS Trust	Yes	Yes
University Hospitals of Morecambe Bay NHS Trust	Yes	Yes
Walsall Hospitals NHS Trust	Yes	No
West Hertfordshire Hospitals NHS Trust	No	No
West Middlesex University Hospital NHS Trust	No	No
West Suffolk Hospitals NHS Trust	Yes	Yes
Whipps Cross University Hospital NHS Trust	Yes	Yes
Whittington Hospital NHS Trust	Yes	Yes
Winchester & Eastleigh Healthcare NHS Trust	Yes	Yes
Wirral Hospital NHS Trust	Yes	Yes
Worcestershire Acute Hospitals	Yes	Yes
Worthing and Southlands Hospitals NHS Trust	Yes	Yes
Wrightington, Wigan & Leigh NHS Trust	Yes	Yes
Yeovil District Hospital NHS Foundation Trust	Yes	Yes
York Hospitals NHS Trust	Yes	Yes

Trusts are listed that were expected to participate.

APPENDIX G - Corporate structure

The National Confidential Enquiry into Patient Outcome and Death (NCEPOD) is an independent body to which a corporate commitment has been made by the Medical and Surgical Colleges, Associations and Faculties related to its area of activity. Each of these bodies nominates members on to NCEPOD's Steering Group.

Steering Group as at 21st November 2007

Dr D Whitaker	Association of Anaesthetists of Great Britain and Ireland
Mr T Bates	Association of Surgeons of Great Britain & Ireland
Dr S Bridgman	Faculty of Public Health Medicine
Dr P Cartwright	Royal College of Anaesthetists
Dr P Nightingale	Royal College of Anaesthetists
Dr B Ellis	Royal College of General Practitioners
Ms M McElligott	Royal College of Nursing
Prof D Luesley	Royal College of Obstetricians and Gynaecologists
Mrs M Wishart	Royal College of Ophthalmologists
Dr I Doughty	Royal College of Paediatrics and Child Health
Dr R Dowdle	Royal College of Physicians
Professor T Hendra	Royal College of Physicians
Dr M Armitage	Royal College of Physicians
Dr M Clements	Royal College of Physicians
Dr A Nicholson	Royal College of Radiologists
Mr B Rees	Royal College of Surgeons of England
Mr M Parker	Royal College of Surgeons of England
Mr D Mitchell	Faculty of Dental Surgery, Royal College of Surgeons of England
Dr S Lishman	Royal College of Pathologists
Ms S Panizzo	Patient Representative
Mrs M Wang	Patient Representative

Observers

Mrs C Miles	Institute of Healthcare Management
Dr R Palmer	Coroners' Society of England and Wales
Mrs H Burton	Scottish Audit of Surgical Mortality
Mrs E Stevenson	National Patient Safety Agency

Dr K Cleary National Patient Safety Agency

NCEPOD is a company, limited by guarantee and a registered charity, managed by Trutees.

Trustees

Clinical Co-ordinators

The Steering Group appoint a Lead Clinical Co-ordinator for a defined tenure. In addition there are seven Clinical Co-ordinators who work on each study. All Co-ordinators are engaged in active academic/clinical practice (in the NHS) during their term of office.

Lead Clinical Co-ordinator Mr I C Martin (Surgery)

Clinical Co-ordinators Dr D G Mason (Anaesthesia)
Dr J Stewart (Medicine)
Professor S B Lucas (Pathology)
Dr G Findlay (Intensive Care)
Dr D Mort (Medicine)
Mr S Carter (Surgery)
Mr M Lansdown (Surgery)